GET FIT FOR YOUR HOLIDAY in 28 days

Heather Bampfylde

COLLINS

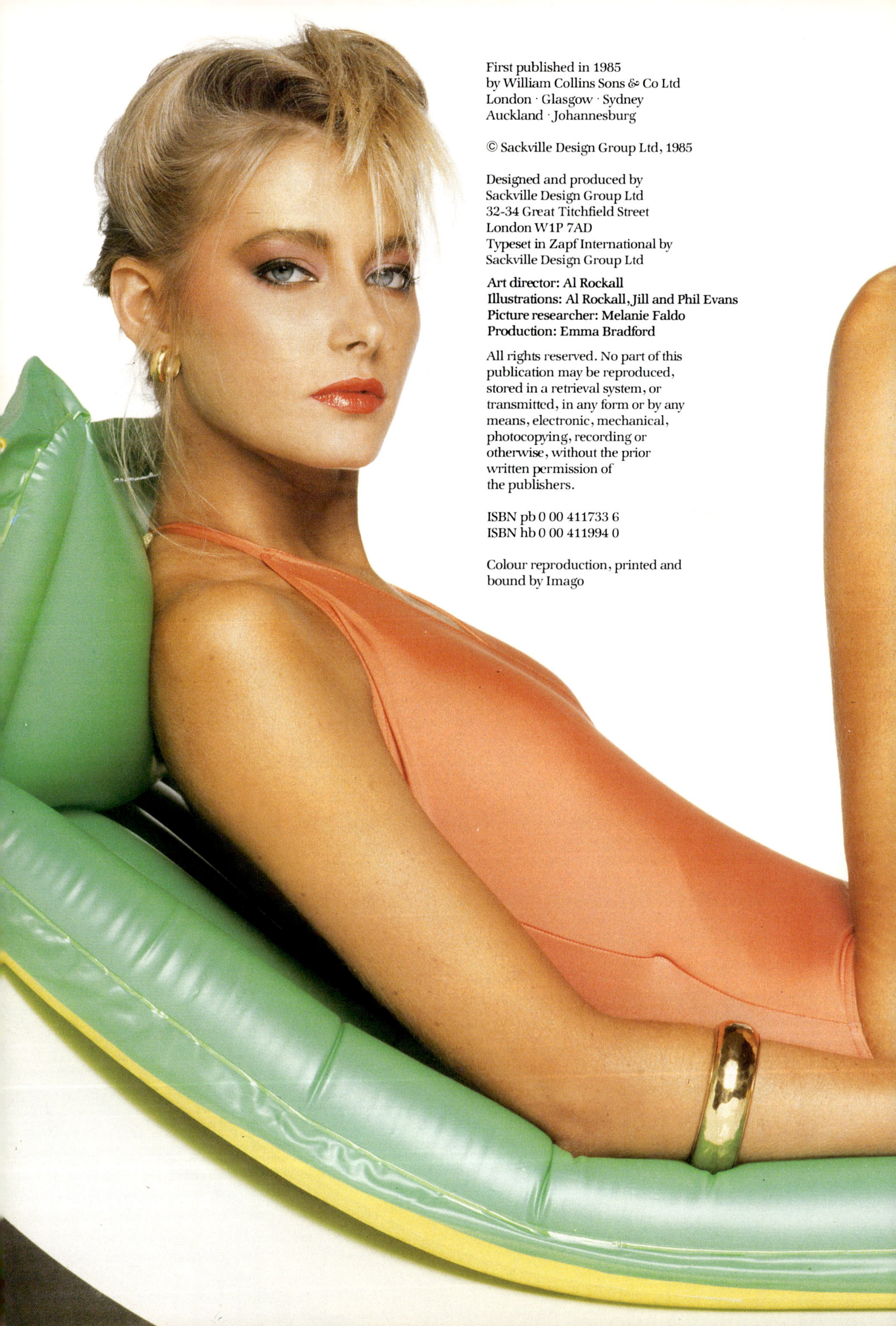

First published in 1985
by William Collins Sons & Co Ltd
London · Glasgow · Sydney
Auckland · Johannesburg

Designed and produced by
Sackville Design Group Ltd
32-34 Great Titchfield Street
London W1P 7AD
Typeset in Zapf International by
Sackville Design Group Ltd

Art director: Al Rockall
Illustrations: Al Rockall, Jill and Phil Evans
Picture researcher: Melanie Faldo
Production: Emma Bradford

ISBN pb 0 00 411733 6
ISBN hb 0 00 411994 0

Colour reproduction, printed and bound by Imago

GET FIT FOR YOUR HOLIDAY *in 28 days*

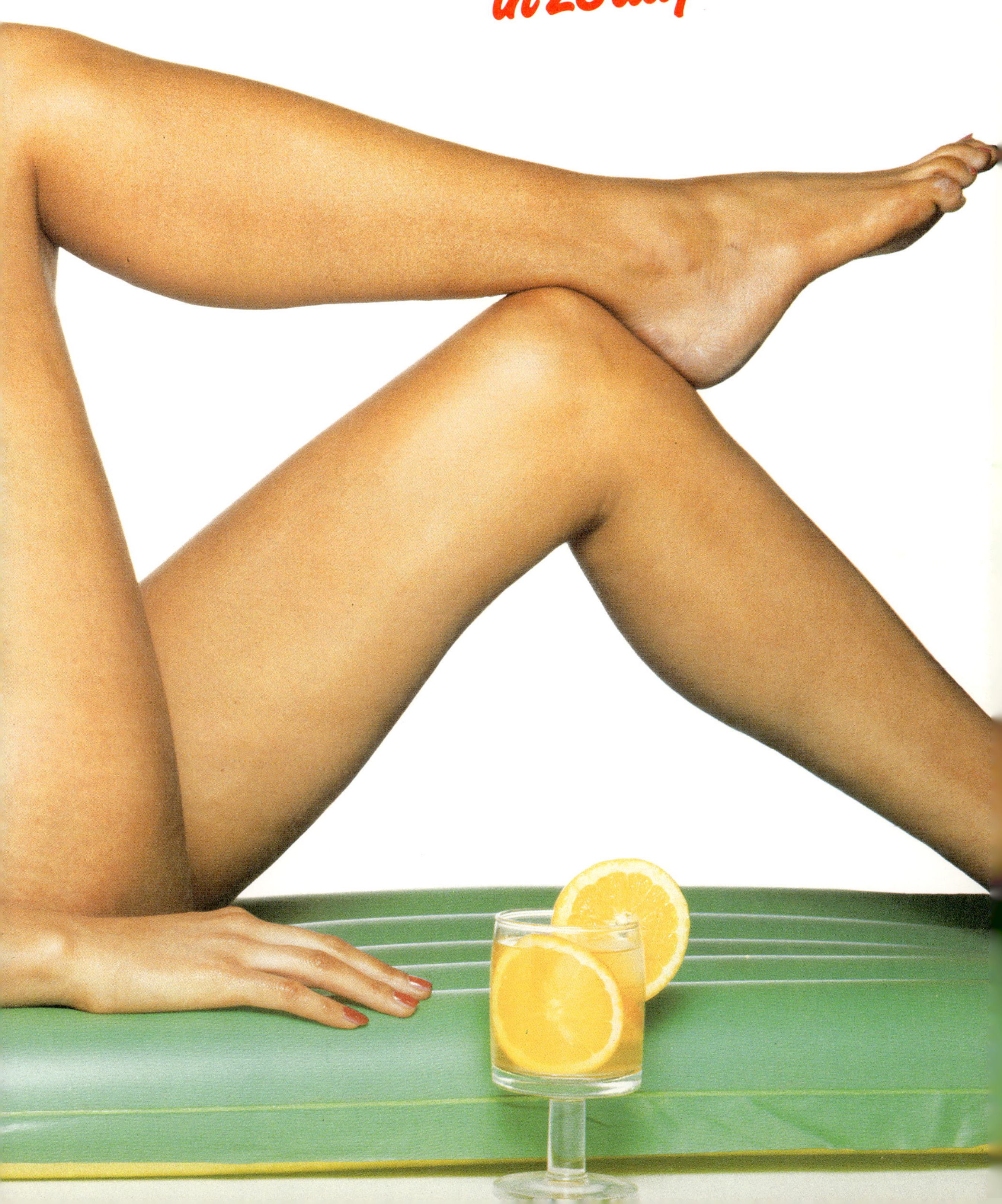

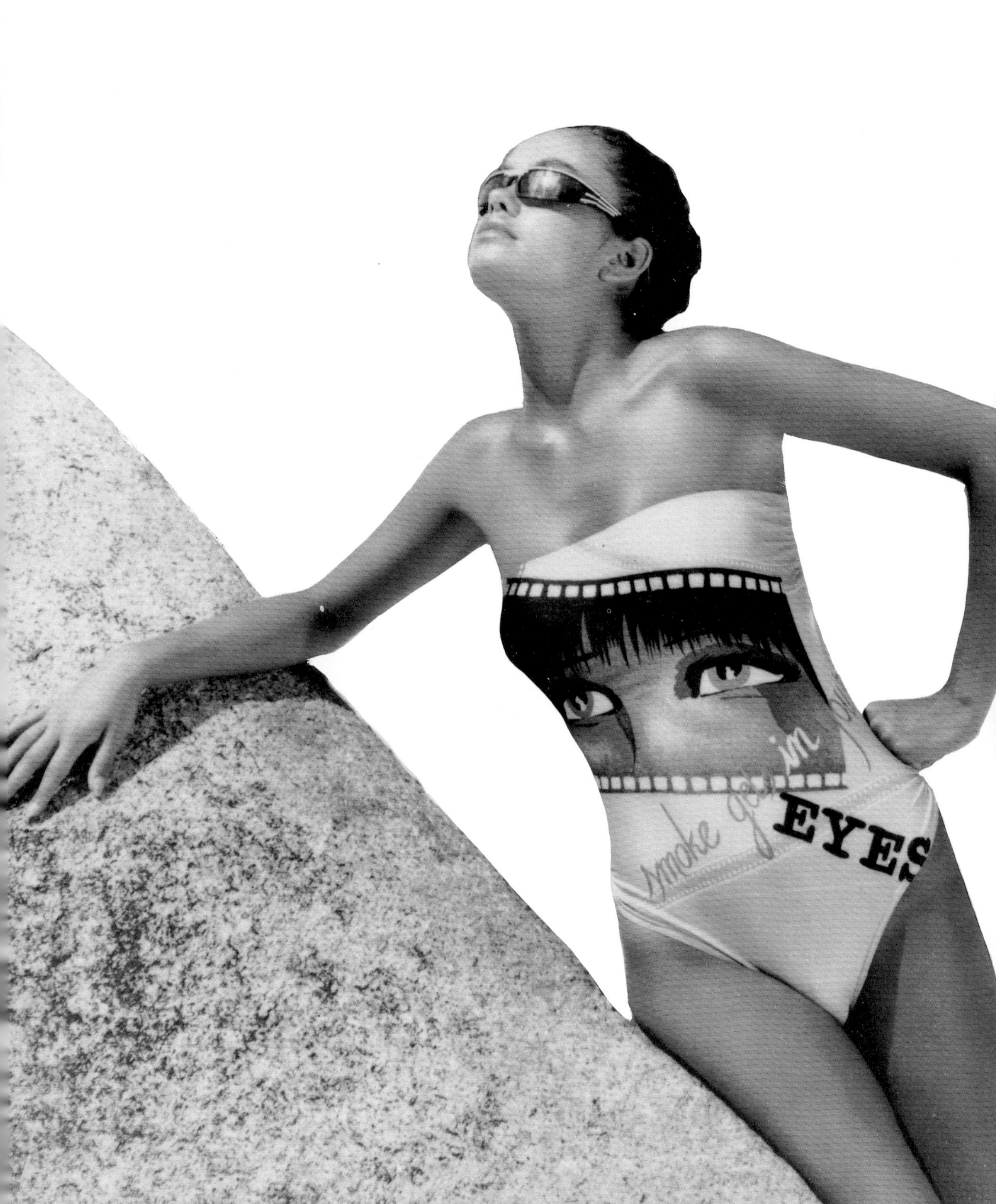
EYES

Contents

Introduction	6
Your 28-day diet plan	8
Your 28-day exercise programme	14
Days 1-7	16
Holiday suncare	30
Days 8-14	32
Holiday haircare	46
Days 15-21	48
Holiday make-up	62
Days 22-28	64
Holiday checklist	78
Choosing the right holiday	80
Travelling light	82
Your health	84
Keep fit on holiday	86
Motoring abroad	88
Money	90
Adventure holidays	91
Air travel	92
Index	94

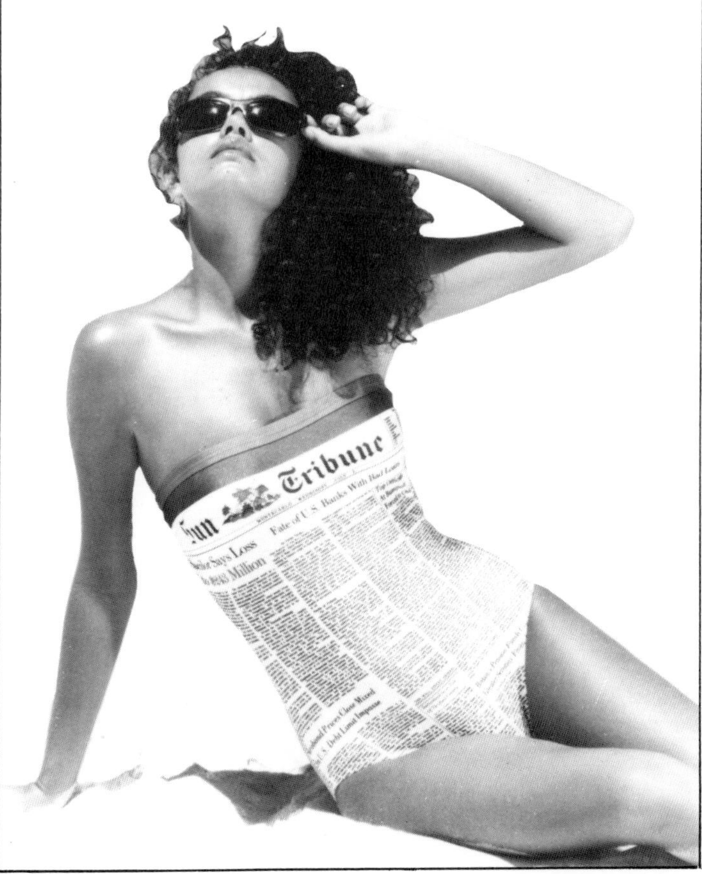

Your guide to holiday health and beauty

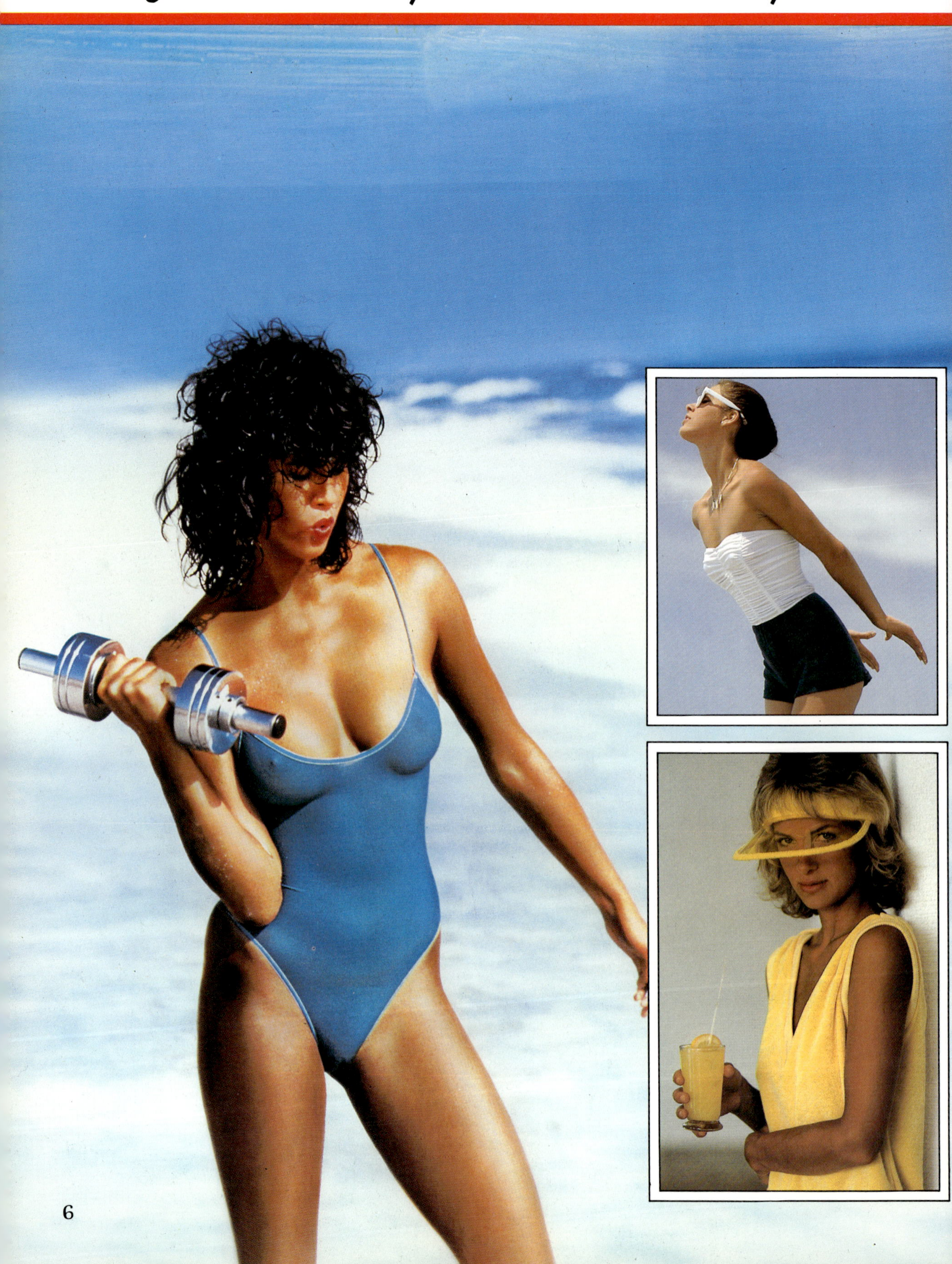

Introduction

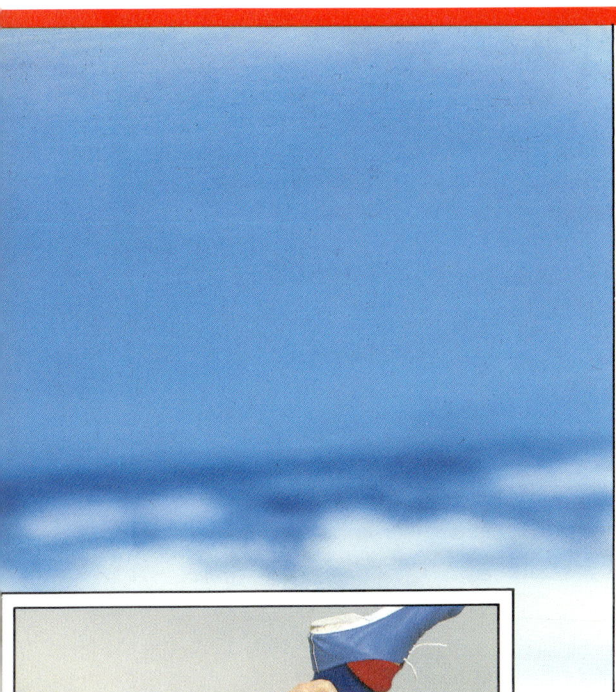

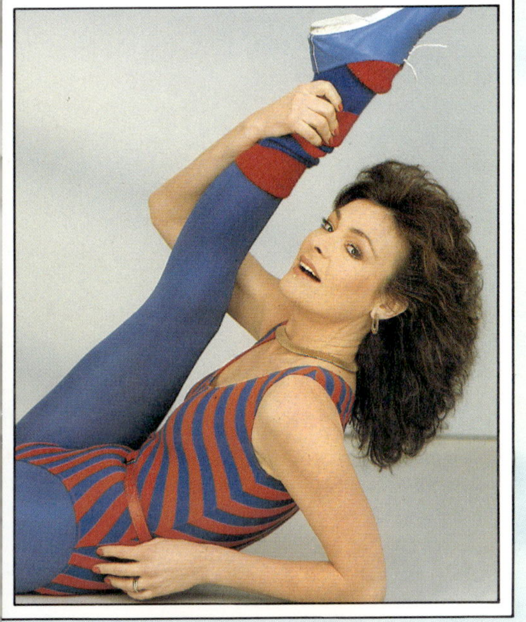

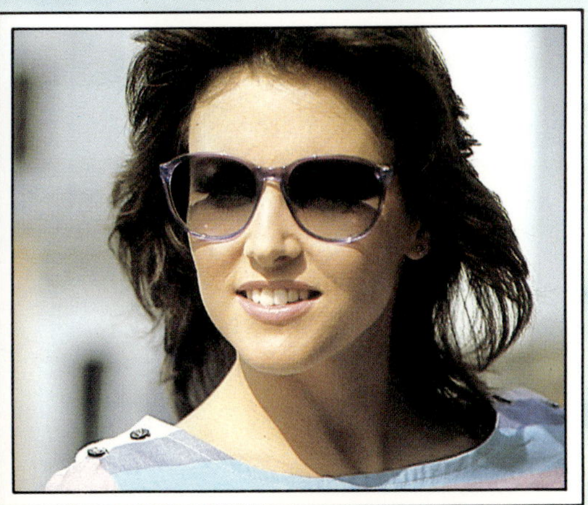

This comprehensive beauty, health and fitness package offers you a unique day-by-day guide to getting holiday-ready. It tells you how to get fit and slim for the beach and the sunshine. By following it in the weeks leading up to your departure date, you can prepare your skin in readiness for a holiday tan, shed any excess weight, firm up slack muscles, work on reducing any flabby areas, and make sure that your body looks good in a swimsuit.

In order to make the programme work for you, it is important to make time for yourself, no matter how busy you are. The daily beauty, exercise and diet guidelines are not mere self-indulgence — on the contrary, they are essential for your long-term health and well-being. If you want to look your best, you have to spend time on the basics and make self-care a regular part of everyday living. In 28 days, you can achieve a great deal — equivalent to a two-week stay at a top health farm, and cheaper, too.

All you need do is to follow the day-by-day instructions and advice and you will be amazed at how much better you look and feel. Learn how to eat a really healthy wholefoods diet to lose weight, spring-clean your body and make your hair *and* skin more beautiful. This means cutting out processed convenience foods and enjoying the real flavours and textures of fresh ingredients, confident that they are doing you good.

Good diet alone will not make you fit and slim, so you will need to supplement it with daily exercise to tone up your muscles and give you a really slim summer shape. You can choose from several aerobic sports and exercises in addition to following our great all-over body work-out. Of course, your figure and degree of fitness at the end of the programme will depend to some extent on your physical shape and condition at the beginning and how religiously you stick to the guidelines. If you are reasonably active and slim before you start, you will probably be fitter on Day 28 than someone who is overweight and unused to exercise. However, even these women can benefit enormously from the programme and can revolutionise their lives by stepping up their activity level and eating a healthy diet.

The beauty regime will help you develop good skin and haircare habits by providing you with the know-how and lots of practical expert advice. You are shown how to develop a glorious tan the easy, painless way and how to prepare your skin even before you leave home. You can learn the secrets of beauty on the beach and how to make-up for the sun and sea.

The programme is not easy and you may find it difficult in the first week to fit all the extra activities, exercise and beauty routines into your normal schedule, but these weeks of preparation will pay off and help you to enjoy your holiday even more than usual. Make this a memorable holiday by capitalising on your new-found fitness and good looks so that you enjoy being outside in the warm sunshine and getting away from it all.

Your 28-day diet plan

This diet will help you lose excess weight and feel fitter and healthier for your holiday. It will spring-clean your body and promote lasting health and beauty. Low in calories and high in nutritional goodness, it is based on fresh wholefood ingredients — vegetables, fruit, whole grain bread and cereals, fish, chicken and yoghurt.

It is quick and easy to prepare, inexpensive if you live on a tight budget and varied enough to prevent boredom setting in. It is sufficiently flexible to allow you some degree of choice at every meal — whether it's breakfast, lunch or dinner. Unlike many faddy diets (for example, cottage cheese and grapefruit only regimes), it includes a wide range of foods, and there is a delicious Dish of the Day suggested for most of the 28 days if you are stuck for ideas. In fact, the food is so good and healthy that the rest of the family won't mind sharing it.

Fibre

Nutritionists and doctors now recognise that fibre plays an important part in promoting good health and the prevention of many modern diseases. It also helps you to lose weight by speeding up the passage of food through your body, preventing constipation and filling you up so that you do not want to eat so many sweet and high-calorie foods. A high-fibre diet has beauty spin-offs, too, as it removes toxic waste-products from your body. Thus you will have clearer skin and more glossy hair. Most fresh fruit and vegetables, beans and pulses and whole grains are a good source of fibre. Always eat 100 per cent wholemeal (not white) bread, and opt for brown rice and muesli rather than white rice or sweetened commercial breakfast cereals.

Protein

You will notice that there may seem to be less protein in this diet than the amounts you are used to eating. Most of us eat more protein than our bodies need, especially red meats (beef, lamb and pork) and hard cheeses which contain saturated fats. In this diet, you can choose between white fish, chicken, low-fat cheese, eggs and skimmed milk as sources of protein. Don't forget vegetable protein which is equally important — that is why you can eat plenty of whole grain bread, jacket potatoes, brown rice and beans.

Packed lunches

If you go out to work you can take a packed lunch with you. Don't make working an excuse for skipping your diet. You can prepare a delicious salad with fresh fruit, yoghurt and wholemeal bread and take it with you in an airtight container. Put it in the refrigerator at work if there is one to keep it cool and fresh in hot weather. If you leave home early prepare it the night before.

Diet rules

In order to lose weight and enjoy the beauty benefits of this diet you *must* observe the following rules:

1 Reduce your salt intake. Sprinkle less on your food, and try out fresh herbs and spices as more healthy seasonings. By cutting out processed foods your salt intake will drop significantly.
2 No sugar — and that means sugarless drinks, no cakes, biscuits, sweets and sugary desserts or sweetened yoghurts. Not only will you get slimmer and stay that way by breaking the sugar habit, but you will also require less visits to the dentist.
3 Cut down on fats by eliminating butter and cream from your diet. Choose skimmed rather than whole milk; low-fat soft cheeses (not hard ones) like cottage, ricotta, quark and fromage frais; pure vegetable margarines if you really must spread something on your bread, but only a scraping; and grill rather than fry/roast fish and chicken.
4 No soft, fizzy drinks — mineral water is healthier and has no calories.
5 Reduce your alcohol consumption to a maximum of one glass of white wine a day — or better still, cut it out altogether. Not only will you feel healthier and more energetic — you will look better too, with brighter eyes and glowing, clear skin.
6 Cut down on caffeine by giving up coffee. Try a caffeine-free substitute — most supermarkets now sell their own brand. Even tea contains some caffeine so you could try going without that, too. Try some of the delicious herbal teas available from health food shops.
7 Definitely *no* processed or convenience foods. The list of prohibited foods includes potato crisps, salted peanuts, all canned and packaged foods, chocolates, sweets, processed meats and cheeses. Most are high in unwanted calories, sugar, salt and additives.
8 And now for the positive side — eat plenty of fresh fruit and vegetables, especially in their raw state. Always remember to wash them first to remove traces of any poisonous sprays.
9 No sweet puddings — have fresh fruit or unsweetened natural yoghurt instead. They are more healthy and tend to be lower in calories.
10 Make sure you eat plenty of high-fibre foods.

The diet

Here are the diet guidelines for breakfast, lunch and dinner with suggested snacks if you really can't resist the temptation to eat between meals. For the sake of your holiday figure, however, and the bikini you aspire to wear on the beach, make a special effort to eat only those foods that are permitted if you wish to lose weight.

Breakfast choices

Choose one of the following:

1 Small helping unsweetened muesli (see recipe) with skimmed milk or natural unsweetened yoghurt and fruit of your choice

2 Dried fruit (apricots, peaches, prunes, apples etc.) soaked overnight in lemon juice and water
3 One egg, poached or boiled, with one slice 100 per cent wholemeal bread/toast with a scraping of vegetable margarine (optional)
4 150ml/5floz unsweetened natural yoghurt with bran and wheatgerm and chopped fresh fruit of your choice (banana, apple, orange, berry fruits, peach etc.)
5 150ml/5floz unsweetened natural yoghurt whizzed up in a blender with 1 banana or slice fresh pineapple, skimmed milk and brewers yeast powder plus dash of vanilla extract
6 Half grapefruit, with one slice 100 per cent wholemeal bread/toast with scraping of vegetable margarine (optional) or 2 oatcakes
7 Fresh orange and grapefruit salad (peeled and sliced in own juice), with 1 slice wholemeal bread/toast
plus one of the following breakfast drinks:
1 Unsweetened fruit or vegetable juice of your choice
2 Hot water mixed with juice of half a lemon
3 Herbal tea or decaffeinated coffee or unsweetened lemon tea

Lunch choices
Choose one of the following:
1 100g/4oz cottage cheese, ricotta, quark or fromage frais
2 75g/3oz chicken or fish, cold or grilled or poached
3 Omelette made with 2 eggs flavoured with fresh herbs, shrimps, tomato, fromage frais or spinach (do not have omelette if you had an egg for breakfast)
4 Dish of the Day if savoury
plus
Unlimited salad of your choice served with a yoghurt dressing (see recipe). Choose from lettuce, Chinese leaves, chicory, curly endive, watercress, mustard and cress, raw spinach, peppers, tomatoes, onions, radish,

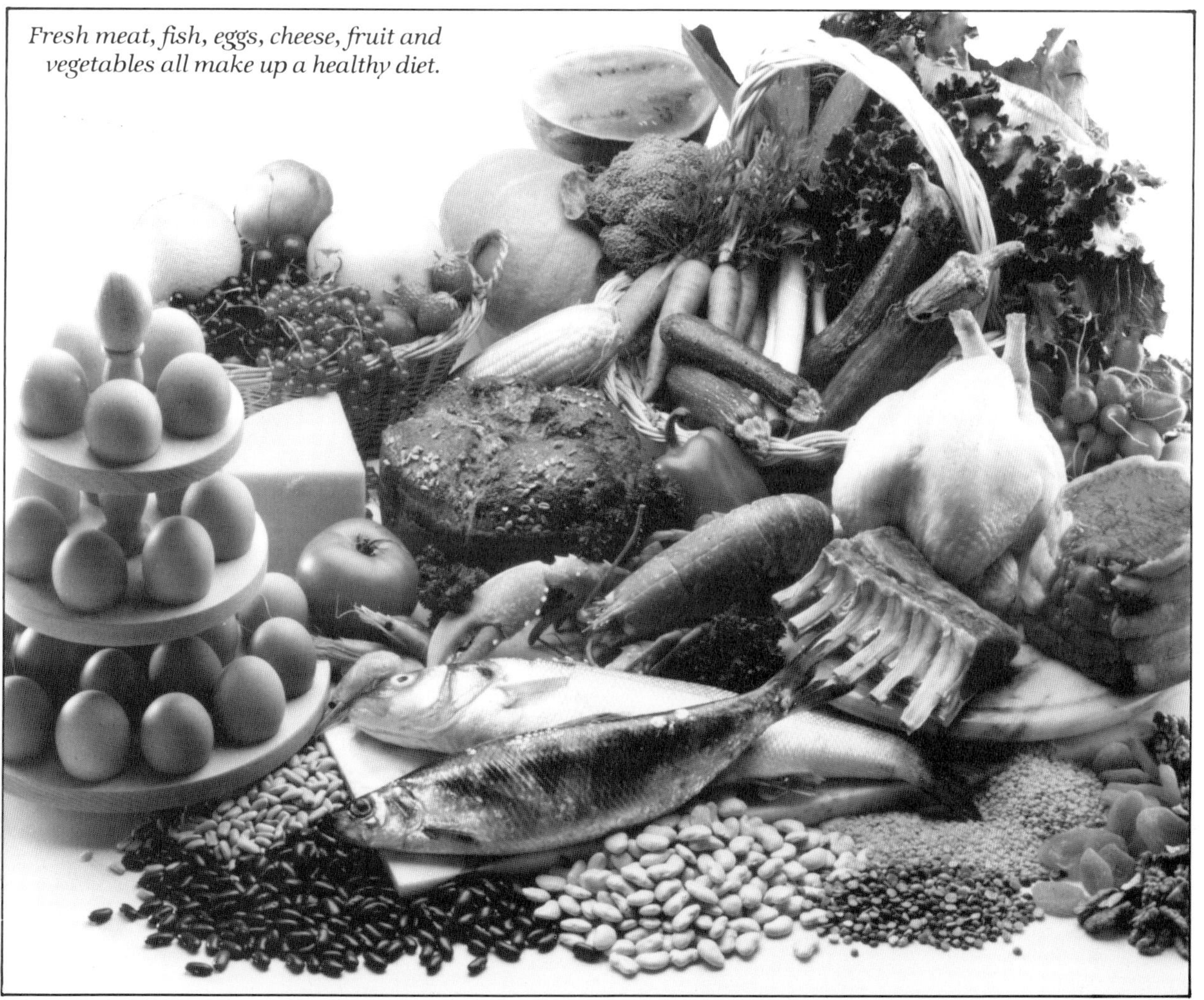

Fresh meat, fish, eggs, cheese, fruit and vegetables all make up a healthy diet.

cucumber, celery, carrot, courgettes, cauliflower florets, mushrooms, alfalfa/bean sprouts
plus
Fresh fruit of your choice
plus
one of the following lunch drinks:
1 Mineral water
2 Herbal tea or decaffeinated coffee or unsweetened lemon tea

Dinner choices
Choose one of the following:
1 75g/3oz chicken or fish, cold or grilled or poached
2 Savoury Dish of the Day (if not eaten at lunchtime)
plus one of the following:
1 Small portion boiled brown rice or wholemeal pasta
2 Slice wholemeal bread
3 Small baked jacket potato topped with a spoonful of natural yoghurt or fromage frais and sprinkling of fresh chopped herbs.
plus one of the following:
1 Fresh fruit
2 Unsweetened natural yoghurt
3 Soft low-fat cheese and celery
4 Sweet Dish of the Day if recipe given
plus one of the following dinner drinks:
1 Mineral water
2 Small glass dry white wine topped up with sparkling mineral water

Snacks and drinks
Choose from these throughout the day but be sensible and try to limit your consumption:
1 Raw vegetable sticks, eg. peppers, carrots, celery
2 Fresh fruit
3 Sunflower, sesame, pumpkin seeds
4 Mineral water

Note: Plan your daily diet in such a way that you vary the food choices and always include at least one slice of 100 per cent wholemeal bread. The Dish of the Day can be substituted if wished at any suitable meal but eaten only once on any day.

Losing weight
The amount of weight you lose will depend on how much you weighed before you started the diet, but most people can expect to lose about 3.5kg/7lb by the end of the 28 day programme. Gradual weight loss is the safest way to slim and eating such healthy food is bound to make you feel and look better before you leave for your holiday. If you are planning on going abroad, especially to the Mediterranean countries, you will probably find that the local diet is very healthy, too. If you eat out away from the main tourist areas, fresh vegetables, fish and white meat often cooked with olive oil, fruit and soft cheeses, and even yoghurt are the normal everyday fare.

If you are already very overweight then your overall weight loss may be more dramatic — even up to 7kg/14lb if you stick religiously to the diet guidelines. Don't spoil all the good work by guzzling too many cream cakes, ice-creams and other fattening foods while you're away. Try to keep your new slim figure by continuing with your healthy eating habits. Obviously, there will be occasional lapses when you go out to dinner and can't resist a dessert off the sweets trolley or you crave for a bar of chocolate but keep these for special occasions.

Meanwhile, here are a few basic recipes which you may find helpful and an essential part of your new healthy diet. If you do not have the time or inclination to make your own wholemeal bread and live yoghurt, you can buy these at most health food stores. And even some bakeries now make 100 per cent wholemeal bread without any additives.

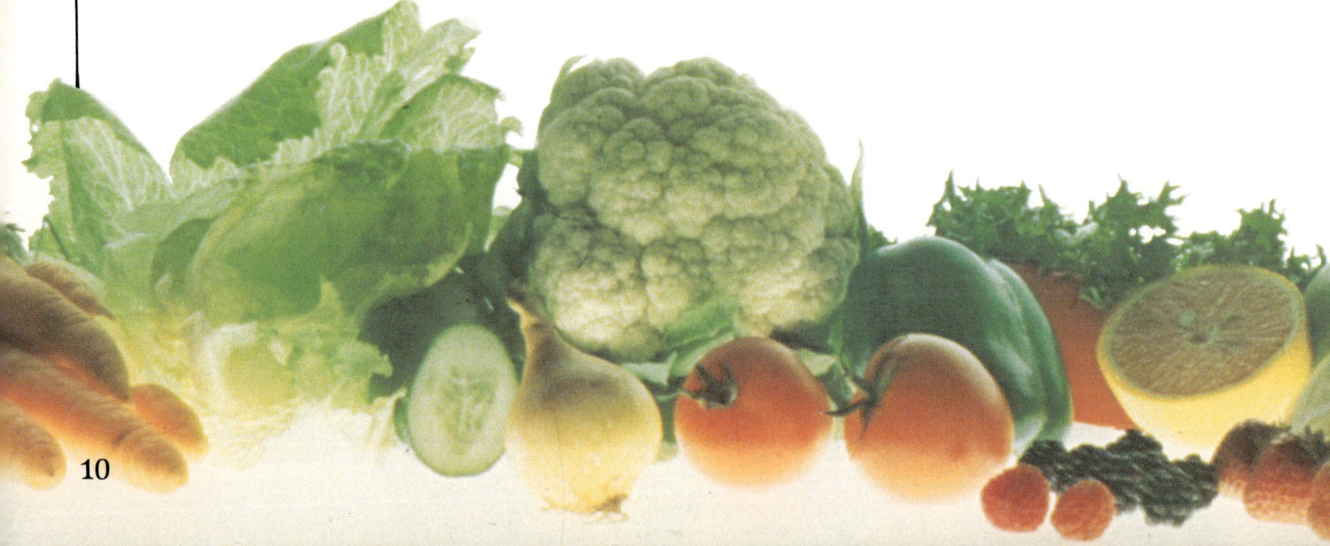

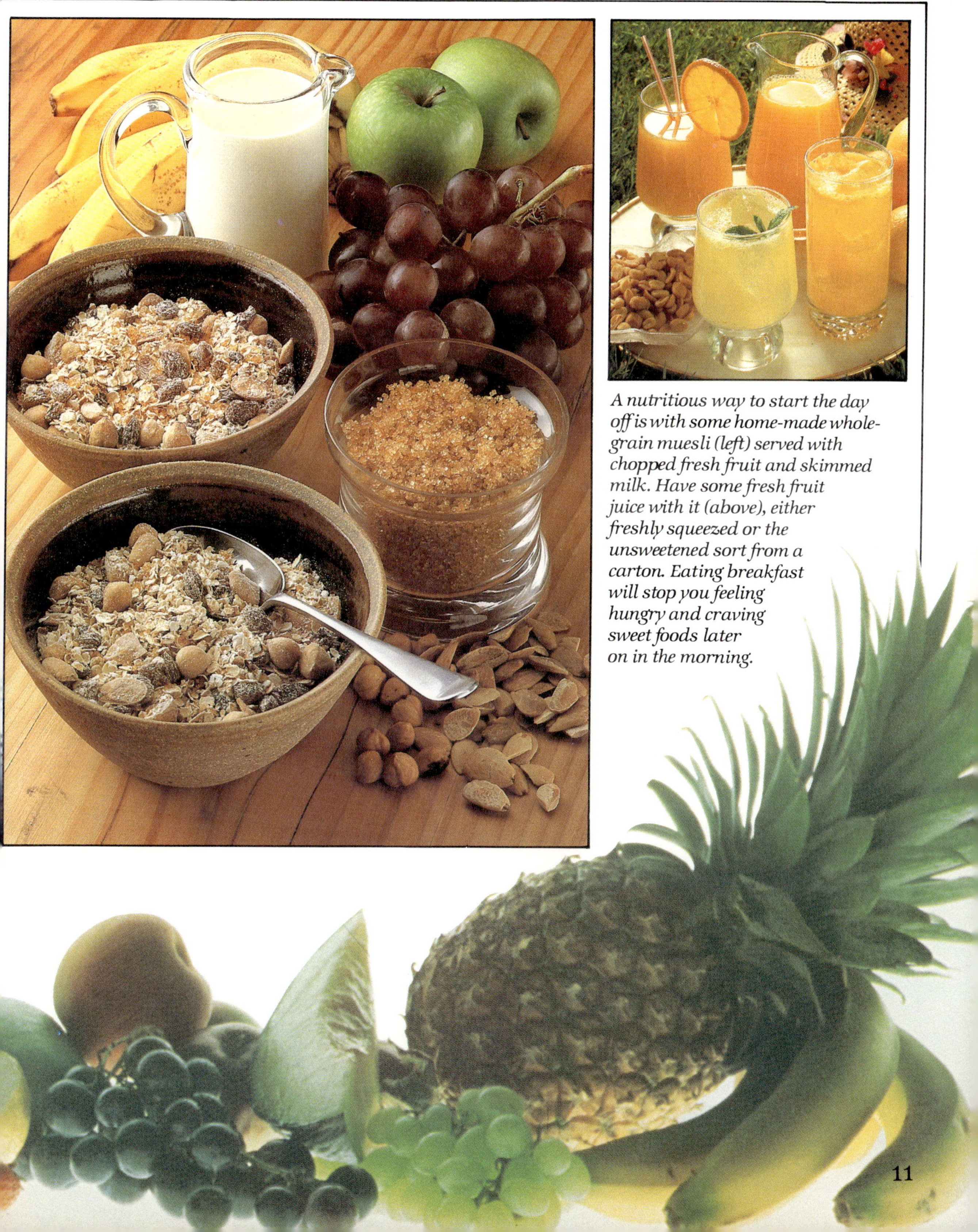

A nutritious way to start the day off is with some home-made whole-grain muesli (left) served with chopped fresh fruit and skimmed milk. Have some fresh fruit juice with it (above), either freshly squeezed or the unsweetened sort from a carton. Eating breakfast will stop you feeling hungry and craving sweet foods later on in the morning.

Quick wholemeal bread
550g/1lb 4oz 100 per cent wholemeal flour
10ml/2 level teaspoons sea salt
1 packet easy blend dried yeast, eg. Harvest Gold
30ml/2 tablespoons vegetable oil
300ml/½ pint water at blood heat
30ml/2 tablespoons molasses
Optional flavourings:
60ml/4 tablespoopns cracked wheat
100g/4oz chopped walnuts
1 small onion, chopped
fresh herbs (parsley, chives, oregano, basil, thyme etc), chopped
1 clove garlic, crushed

This bread can be made by hand or, better still, in a food processor fitted with the plastic dough blade.
By hand: tip flour and salt into a large mixing bowl and sprinkle in the yeast. Mix well with oil, warm water and molasses until you have a soft sticky dough. Knead well on a floured board until smooth and elastic.
By processor: with machine operating, mix the flour, salt and yeast. Then pour oil, water and molasses through the feed tube and process until dough is smooth and elastic and leaves sides of the bowl clean — the action of the processor does all the kneading for you! Shape kneaded dough into a round, place in a well-oiled bowl and tie up in a clean plastic bag. Leave in a warm place for about 1 hour until well-risen and doubled in size. Knock back dough on a floured board and add flavourings of your choice. Knead lightly and shape into loaves. Place in greased loaf tins and leave in warm place until dough rises to the top of tins. Bake in a preheated oven at 230°C/450°F/gas 8 for 25-30 minutes. Cool on a wire rack. Makes 2 small loaves. Can be frozen.

Home-made yoghurt
550ml/1 pint milk
15ml/1 tablespoon skimmed milk powder
30ml/2 tablespoons natural live yoghurt as starter (available from most health food stores)

Mix together milk and skimmed milk powder. Heat until boiling. Remove from heat and cool to 43°C/110-112°F (use a sugar thermometer for accurate reading). Stir the yoghurt starter into the *warm* milk and pour into a *warmed* wide-necked thermos flask or insulated jar. Seal and leave for at least six hours. The yoghurt should be thick, custard-like and pleasantly tart. Transfer to a clean container and refrigerate. Always keep a little of the new yoghurt as a starter for your next batch. Eat on its own or flavour with chopped fresh fruit, wheat germ, bran, muesli, seeds or nuts.

Yoghurt salad dressing
150ml/¼ pint natural yoghurt
juice of ½ lemon
15ml/1 tablespoon finely chopped onion/spring onion
salt and pepper
fresh herbs, chopped
1 crushed clove garlic, optional

Beat all the ingredients together until smooth. Serve with salad at Lunch or Dinner. If wished, add a bunch of washed watercress or a tablespoon of cooked spinach, and blend in a liquidiser or processor.

Breakfast muesli
175g/6oz jumbo oats
50g/2oz rye flakes
25g/1oz bran
25g/1oz raisins
50g/2oz chopped dried dates
25g/1oz chopped hazelnuts
25g/1oz chopped walnuts
25g/1oz chopped cashew/Brazil nuts
25g/1oz chopped dried apricots

Mix all the ingredients together and store in an airtight container. Serve with skimmed milk or yoghurt as directed for Breakfast. Makes 450g/1lb muesli.

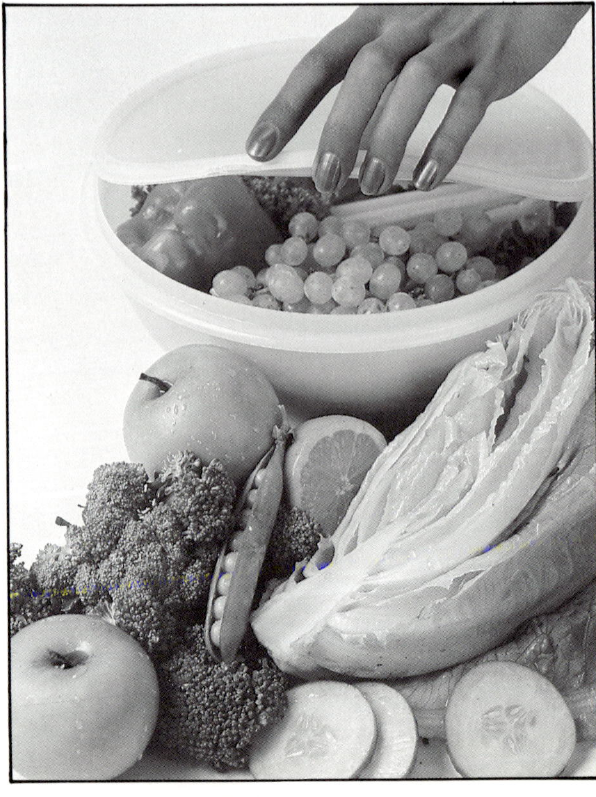

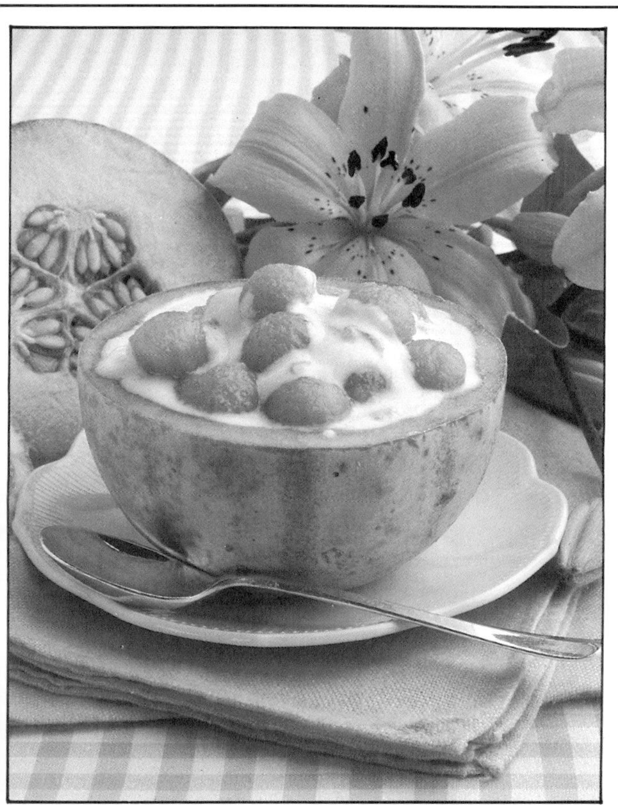

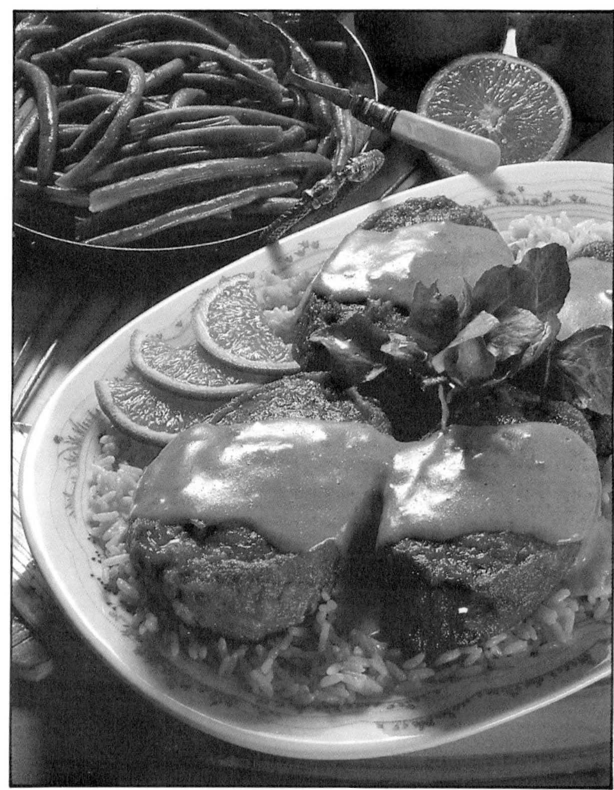

Fresh wholesome foods make delicious healthy and slimming meals. Don't be afraid to experiment with new ideas. A hollowed-out melon filled with juicy melon balls and yoghurt makes a good breakfast or dessert (above), while fish is more tasty served on a bed of rice with a fresh tangy orange and yoghurt sauce (above right).

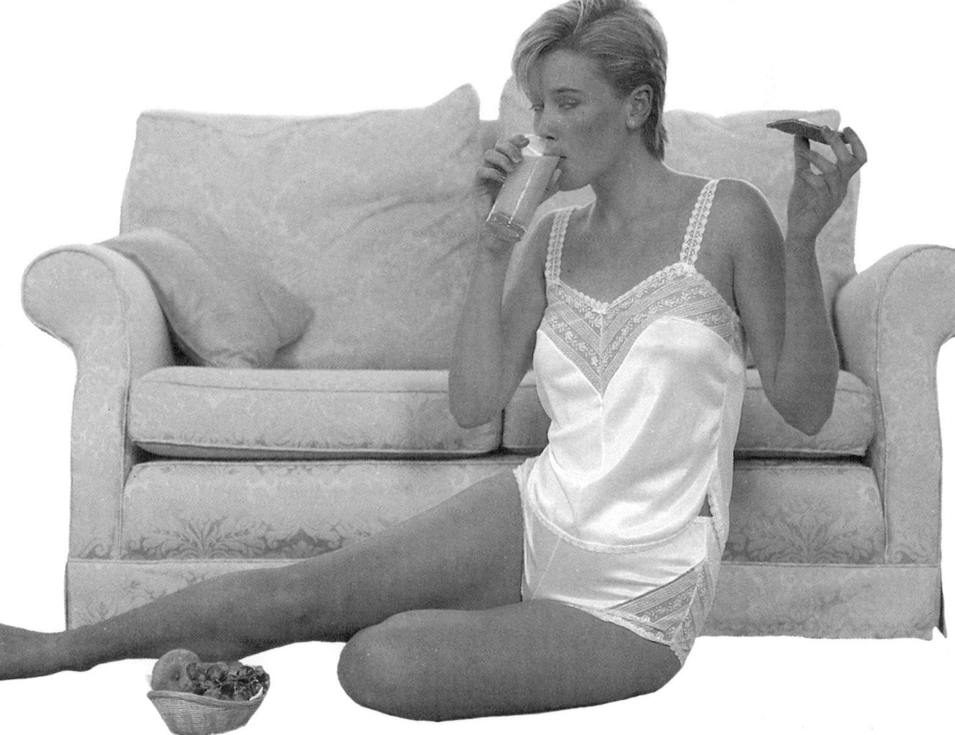

Your 28-day exercise programme

To get fit and slim for your holiday you need to step up your level of exercise. It can be fun and need not be boring or difficult if you start off slowly and build up gently. Even if you are very overweight, you can still slip into a tracksuit and walk or jog. Regular exercise helps you shed excess weight more easily than a crash diet, and if it becomes a part of your daily routine it will ensure that you *stay* slim and healthy.

Your level of fitness at the beginning of the programme will determine what you get out of it. The more unfit you are, the more you stand to gain. But if you have difficulty touching your toes, running flat out for a bus or climbing four flights of stairs, you should take it easy, start off slowly and build up gradually.

Remember that fitness takes time and dedication — it cannot be achieved overnight. This programme will help you to progress slowly towards your fitness goals. The combination of different forms of exercise develops all-over fitness — aerobics for strength and endurance, and isotonics for flexibility.

Aerobics

Running, cycling and swimming are all good examples of aerobic activities. They involve the whole body to make you stronger and fitter. Aerobic sports push up your heart rate although oxygen is used at the same rate at it is supplied so that you should never feel breathless or get into oxygen debt. They strengthen your heart and lung systems and develop stamina.

Isotonics

Most work-out and yoga exercises fall into this category. These tend to concentrate on specific areas of the body — one at a time — and make them more supple and stronger. They are usually performed slowly and rhythmically to tone up muscle.

Exercise gear

Always wear the correct clothing to stay comfortable and cool and to avoid injury. This need not be expensive. For the programme you will need the following:

Running: a tracksuit, or old T-shirt/sweatshirt and loose trousers/shorts. Also, a good pair of running shoes which are designed specially to cushion your feet and legs and prevent injury.

Swimming: a swimsuit or bikini and swimcap.

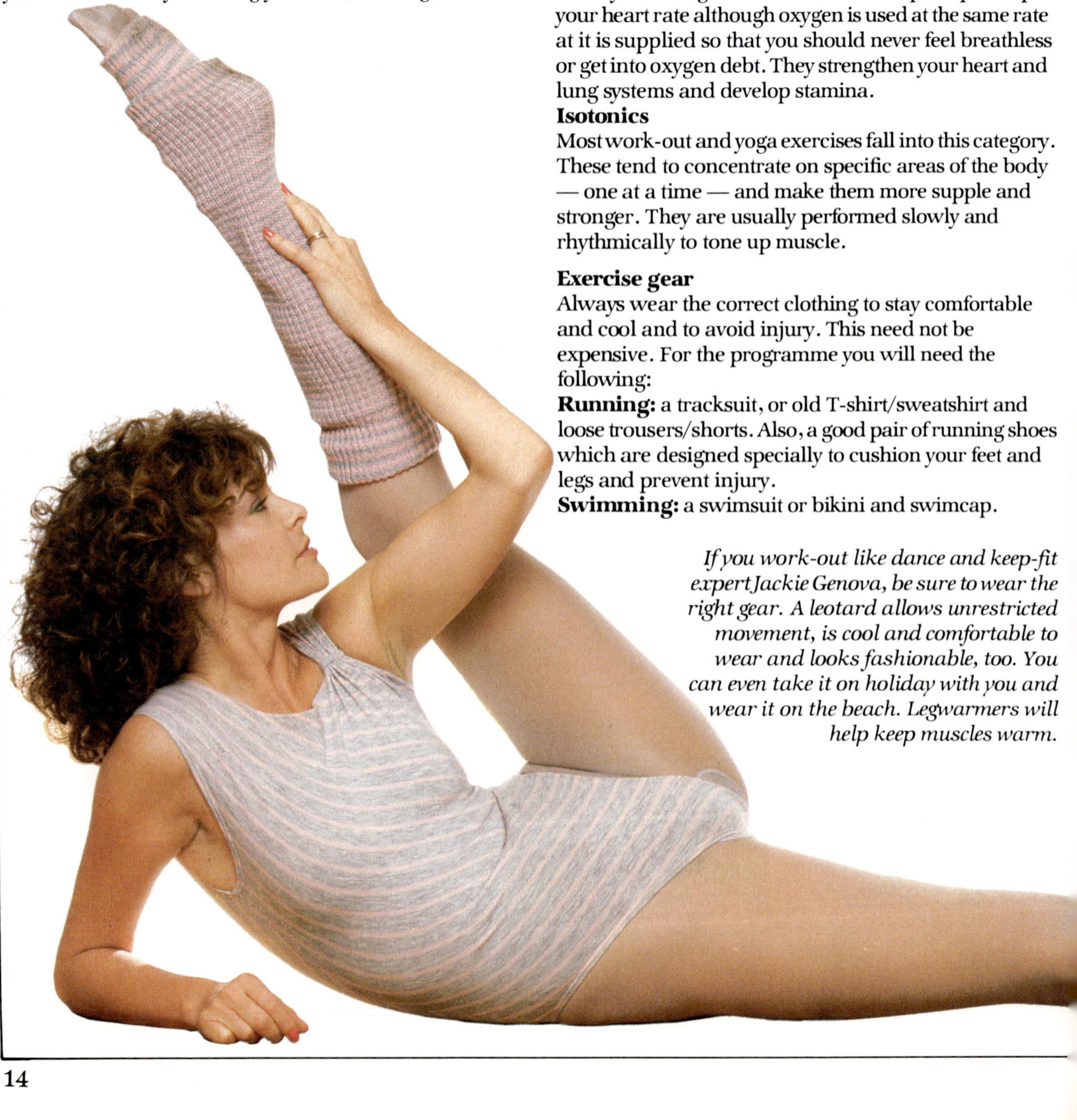

If you work-out like dance and keep-fit expert Jackie Genova, be sure to wear the right gear. A leotard allows unrestricted movement, is cool and comfortable to wear and looks fashionable, too. You can even take it on holiday with you and wear it on the beach. Legwarmers will help keep muscles warm.

Work-out exercises: a leotard or tracksuit or shorts and T-shirt. Legwarmers are a good idea for keeping leg muscles warm and preventing injury.
Cycling: a tracksuit or sweatshirt/T-shirt and loose trousers/shorts plus trainers or your running shoes.
Other sports: for other activities such as tennis, badminton, squash or roller-skating, you will need special equipment and clothing as in the case of tennis rackets, whites and shoes.

Basic exercise guidelines
Whenever you exercise, whether it's running, cycling, yoga or swimming, you should follow these basic guidelines for safety and comfort:

1 Always warm-up first. Use the exercises on page 16.
2 Wear loose, comfortable clothing which will not restrict body movement.
3 Never exercise if you are ill or have a fever.
4 Wait at least one-and-a-half hours after eating.
5 Don't exercise in the hottest part of the day — wait for cooler evening temperatures if the weather is very hot.
6 If an exercise becomes painful, *stop* immediately.
7 Train, don't strain, build up gradually as your level of fitness improves.
8 If you become giddy or dizzy, stop exercising at *once*.
9 Always cool-down after exercising and then relax in a bath or shower.
10 If you are over 35 and have a history of high blood pressure, heart disease or some other serious medical problem, consult your doctor for a complete check-up before embarking on the exercise programme.

At the end of the programme you should be fighting fit and in good shape for your summer bikini — ready to enjoy all the holiday sports and activities on offer. Good luck!

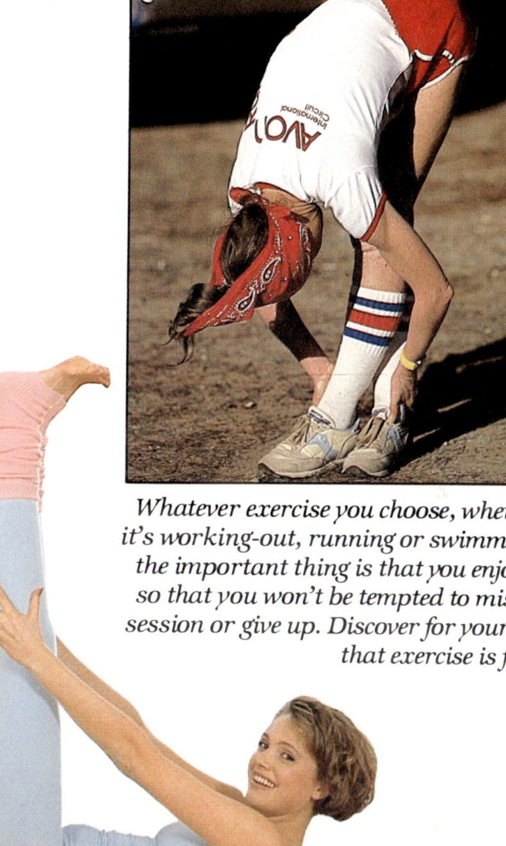

Whatever exercise you choose, whether it's working-out, running or swimming, the important thing is that you enjoy it so that you won't be tempted to miss a session or give up. Discover for yourself that exercise is fun.

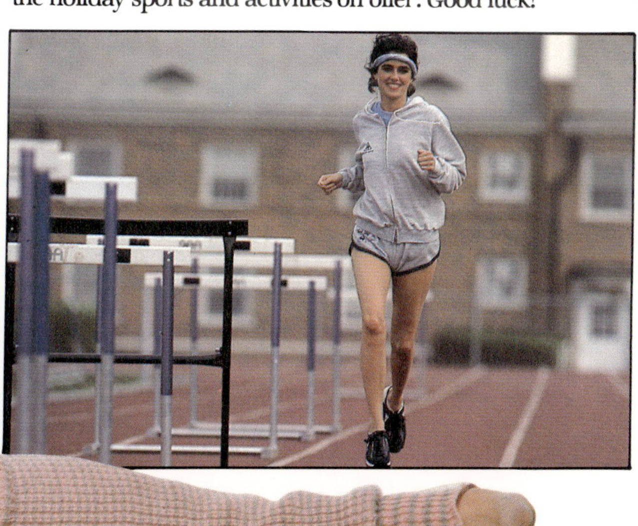

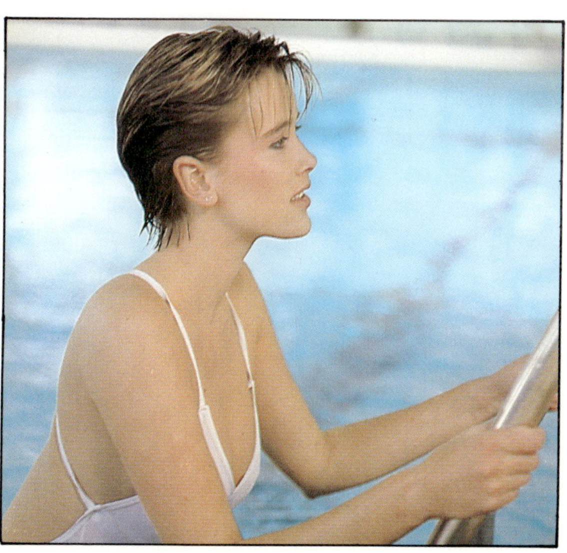

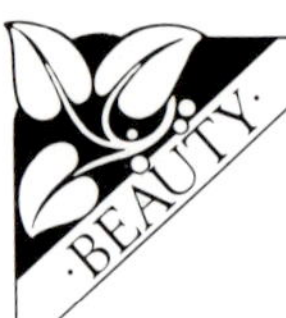

Make up your personal skincare plan

Welcome to the first day of your beauty programme. Start off by inspecting your skin and developing a personal skincare plan. Use a magnifying shaving mirror to check for oiliness, dry patches, blackheads, pimples or wrinkles, and then look at our chart to find out your skin-type and the best way to treat it. All skins, oily, normal or dry, need daily cleansing, toning and moisturising to keep them looking young. So establish a twice-daily routine which will last a lifetime.

Cleanse: every morning, make sure you cleanse with a mild soap, foaming cleanser or milk, cream, oil or lotion, whichever you prefer. This will help keep your skin looking clear and healthy and will unblock pores and remove any impurities.

Tone: next, freshen, or tone, with a fresh, tingly lotion (preferably based on natural ingredients like cucumber or lemon) to stimulate the skin and make it glow.

Moisturise: lastly, moisturise to keep moisture in and make skin smooth, supple and free from lines, dry patches and wrinkles. During the day, a good moisturiser can act as a protective barrier between your skin and the environment.

Repeat the cleanse/tone/moisturise regime in the evening, too — last thing before going to bed. It will remove any dirt, grease or stale make-up and leave skin really clean and able to breathe and renew itself while you are asleep. If you need to buy new beauty products for your skincare programme, always opt for the most natural ones which do not contain harsh chemicals.

Your skincare plan		
Normal skin	Smooth and supple. No shine or enlarged pores. Few blemishes.	Use a mild soap or cleanser, a no-alcohol toner and water-in-oil moisturiser.
Dry skin	Sensitive, flakes easily. Tends to have fine lines and broken capillaries.	Use moisturising cleanser — not soap. Alcohol-free toner and moisturiser, an emollient cream for extra protection.
Oily skin	Shiny, coarse complexion. Large pores and tendency to spots and blackheads.	Wash with soap to cleanse deeply. Tone with slightly astringent lotion. Use oil-absorbing moisturiser.

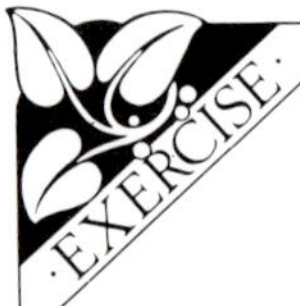

Warm-up and jog

Begin your exercise programme with a few warm-up exercises (shown here) and a jog. Don't neglect the warm-up as this will help stretch out leg muscles and raise your heart rate to pump more oxygen around your body as you run. Aim to run/walk for 15 minutes if you are a complete novice — 20 minutes if you are slightly more experienced. Alternate running and walking as you think fit, and try to run in a relaxed, flowing style using your shoulders to balance you. Use a heel-toe rocking motion, always putting your heel down first to cushion your stride, and pushing off from your toes.

As soon as you feel breathless or uncomfortable, ease down to a gentle jog or walk for a while until you get your breath back and feel more comfortable. Then jog a little way again trying to breathe deeply and easily, running relaxed and easy. Check that there is no tension in your body, that your hands are slightly open (not clenched) and that you are not punching the air. Jogging steadily for just 15 minutes, you can burn up about 150 calories so it is worth persevering for the sake of that holiday swimsuit.

Don't be self-conscious and worry about other people looking at you — runners are now a common sight in most cities and the countryside. Remember to wear loose clothing and running shoes (see page 14). After your run, repeat the stretching exercises to ease out tired muscles and then relax in the bath or a hot shower. The warm water will help fight any muscular stiffness you might feel afterwards.

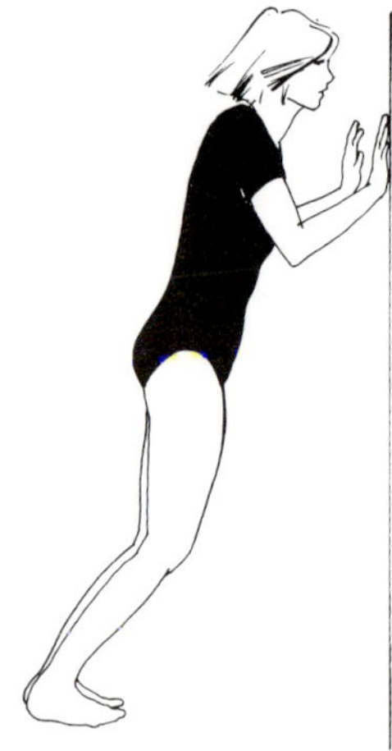

Calf stretch: *this will stretch and ease out your calf muscles before you set out for your run. Lean against a wall or tree with your knees bent and feet about 60cm/2ft away from the wall. Keep your heels firmly on the ground and bend slowly until you feel the stretch in the backs of your legs. Hold for a count of 10. Relax and repeat five times.*

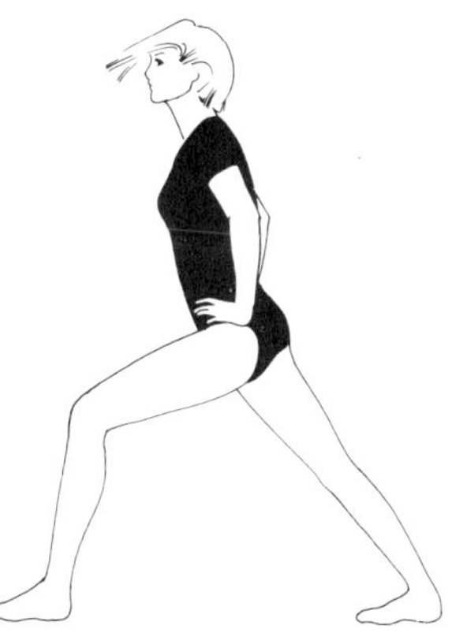

Lunge stretch: *another stretch for calf muscles. Stand with left leg bent facing forwards and right leg outstretched behind you. Your front foot should be as far in front as possible. Hold for a count of 20 and then repeat with the other leg.*

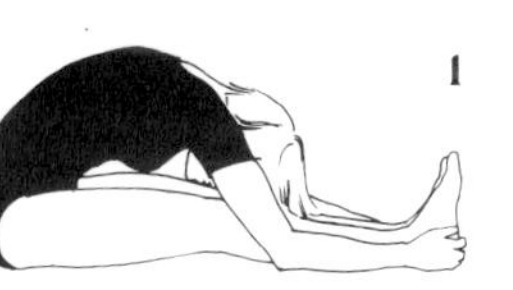

1

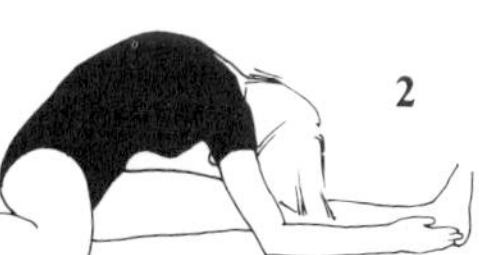

2

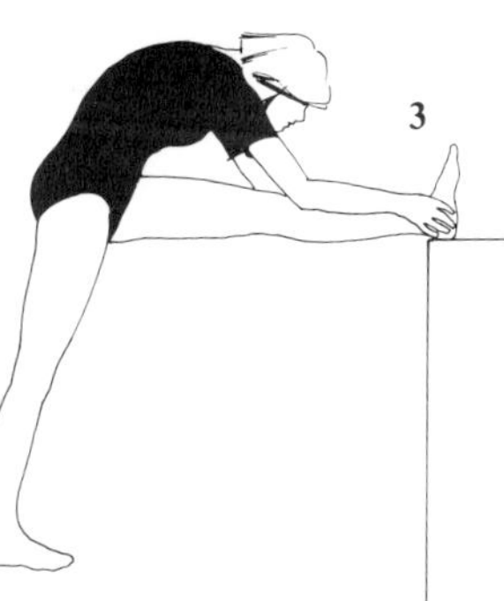

3

Hamstring stretches
1 *Sit bent over your outstretched legs. Hold your heels in your hands and lean forwards as far as you can go — aim to rest your head on your knees. Count to 20.*
2 *Sit with left leg outstretched and right leg bent flat on the floor at 90° angle to your body. Bend over your left leg, clasp your foot and lower head to knee. Hold 30 seconds. Repeat with other leg.*
3 *Rest one leg on support, clasp foot in both hands and lower head to knee. Hold for 30 seconds.*

Holiday tip

Make a resolution to give up smoking *now* or, at least, cut down your daily intake of cigarettes. Smoking interferes with good digestion, constricts tiny blood vessels in your skin, reacts against fitness and may be the cause of many diseases, including chronic bronchitis, lung cancer and heart disease. Give up smoking and you will look, feel and smell better as well as saving much-needed extra money for your holiday. It will be difficult at first but you will soon feel the benefits as the programme progresses and you feel better.

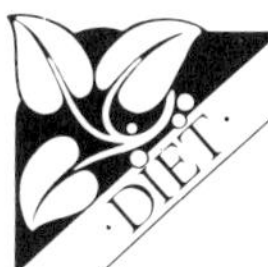

Discover the natural benefits of juice

Throughout the diet programme, you could try making your own fruit and vegetable juices. Freshly squeezed or extracted, they are a rich source of vitamins and minerals with many health and beauty spin-offs. However, they should be drunk immediately after squeezing as their vitamin C content soon diminishes after contact with the air. For fresh citrus drinks — orange, lemon, tangerine or grapefruit — you need only an ordinary squeezer, but for most other fruits and vegetables you will require a juice extractor. These are relatively inexpensive to buy and have far-reaching health benefits. Fresh juices help to cleanse your body of impurities and toxic substances, making your skin and hair look better, too. They are full of nutritional goodness and low in calories so you can drink them with impunity, even on a slimming diet. People with a food processor may be able to buy a special juicer attachment.

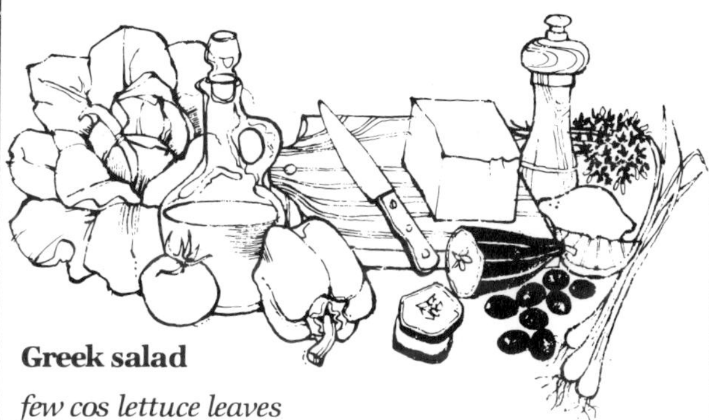

Greek salad

few cos lettuce leaves
2 spring onions, chopped
½ green pepper, sliced
¼ cucumber, sliced
1 tomato, thinly sliced in quarters
15ml/1 tablespoon olive oil
juice ½ lemon
chopped fresh oregano
salt and pepper
75g/3oz Greek feta cheese
few black olives

Mix lettuce, onions, pepper, cucumber and tomato in bowl. Toss in oil and lemon and add oregano and seasoning. Top with thin slices of feta and olives.

Day 2

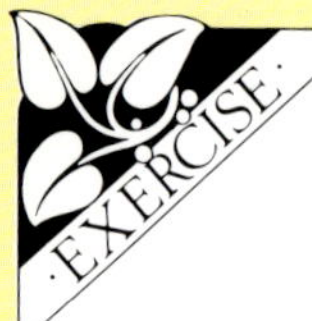

Go for a long walk and work that body!

Go for a good brisk walk today — in the evening or during your lunch break. Or you could even try walking to work or the shops if it's no further than, say, two miles each way. Make walking an integral part of your daily routine. Never get the car out if you can walk instead. It will help burn up calories and make you fitter, especially if you walk at a really brisk pace.

In addition, get going on your home work-out programme. If you have a dance/exercise tape or record which you enjoy, then you can exercise to that. Otherwise, put on a tape with a lively disco beat and try our exercises, working up gradually and doing more repetitions as the programme goes on. Today, concentrate on warm-up exercises and working on your upper body — arms and chest. Upper arms can get very flabby so you will need to work hard to tone up unused muscles and keep them in good shape. Don't worry. These exercises will not develop a rippling muscular physique — it is almost impossible for women to put on the same muscle bulk as men as they do not have the male hormone testosterone.

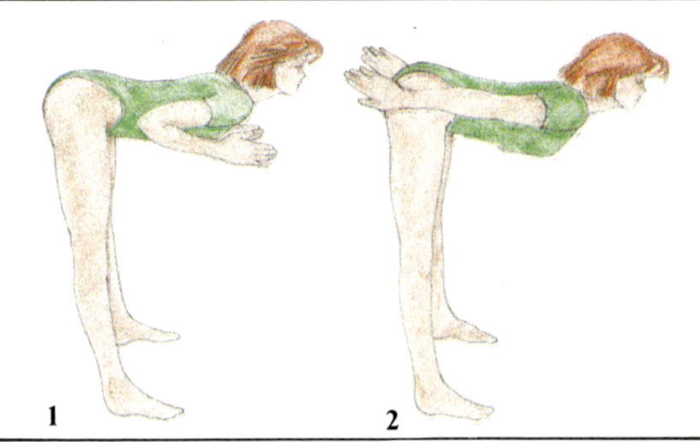

Arm circles
Stand with feet hip distance apart, arms raised above head. Bend arms slightly and circle forwards for 10 counts. Circle backwards for 10 counts ▽

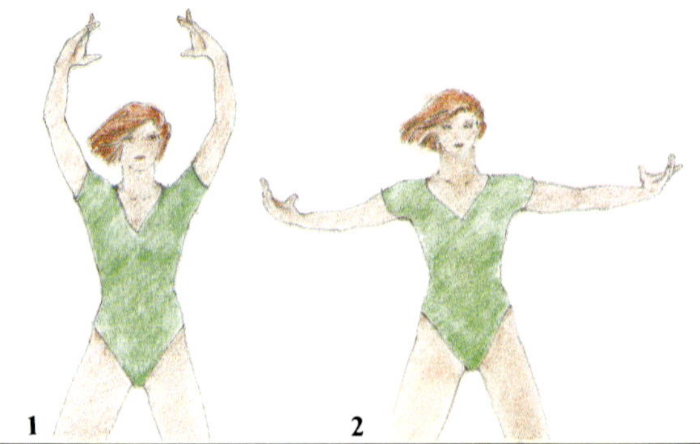

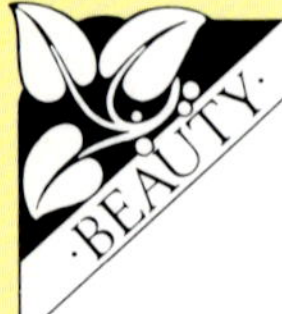

Look after your hair the gentle way

Take a look at your hair today and start working on its condition. Is it dull-looking or shining and glossy? Is it oily or dry? Are the ends split and brittle or neatly cut? By the time you leave for your holiday your hair should be in great condition if you follow the programme. Establishing a proper hair routine is just as important as your skincare, so start today as you mean to continue. Use a shampoo that is specially formulated for your type of hair — dry, normal, oily, permed or bleached. Massage gently into the scalp and then rinse thoroughly. Now apply a conditioner — if your hair is really out of condition, use a special protein pack or hot wax treatment. Leave on the hair for the specified time and then rinse thoroughly. A good conditioner helps protect your hair, giving it smoothness and a healthy shine. Gently comb out any tangles after towelling-dry and then dry your hair in your usual style. Hairdryers are fast but they can damage hair if used wrongly. Hold at least 15cm/6in away from your head and keep moving the dryer around so as not to concentrate the heat for too long on one small area.

If you use heated rollers protect your hair from their drying effects by wrapping some tissue paper around it. Curling tongs are best avoided as these can scorch and damage your hair. Always use this routine whenever you wash your hair — shampoo, rinse, condition, rinse, set and dry. Try shampoos and conditioners based on natural ingredients like scented coconut, apricot oil, avocado, jojoba or herbs. For oily hair, try lemon; for thin, brittle hair, balsam; herbs for dull hair; nettle or seaweed for dandruff; camomile for blondes; henna for brunettes; and protein for damaged hair. A good range of hair products can be found in most health stores.

How often should you wash your hair — whenever it needs shampooing. There is nothing worse than dirty or greasy hair, and it will probably need more frequent washing in hot weather. Be your own judge. Even daily washing cannot harm your hair if done properly with a very mild shampoo. Whereas normal hair will last from five to seven days without washing, greasy hair may need washing after only a couple of days.

Triceps extension
1 *Stand with feet hip distance apart and lean forwards from the waist, keeping your back straight and arms bent, elbows close to the sides.*
2 *Swing your arms back, moving the lower arms only from the elbows down. Swing lower arms forwards and repeat the exercise 20 times.*

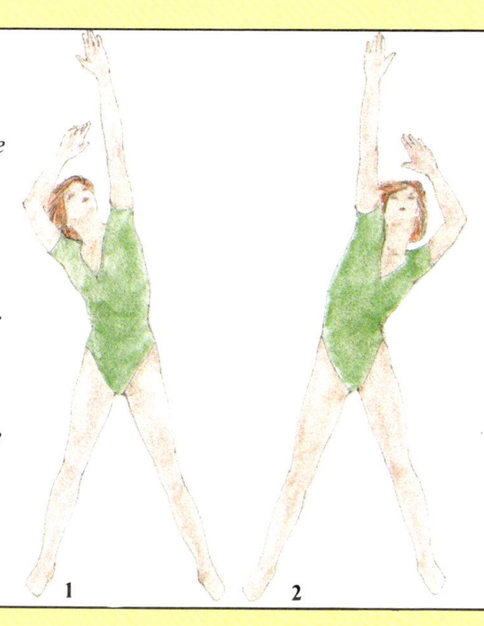

Stretch and bounce warm-up
1 *Breathe in and raise your arms above head, reaching up high with left arm.*
2 *Breathe out and repeat with right arm.*
3 *Lean forwards from waist with straight back and arms outstretched to sides and gently bounce down 4 times.*
4 *Repeat 10 times.* ▽

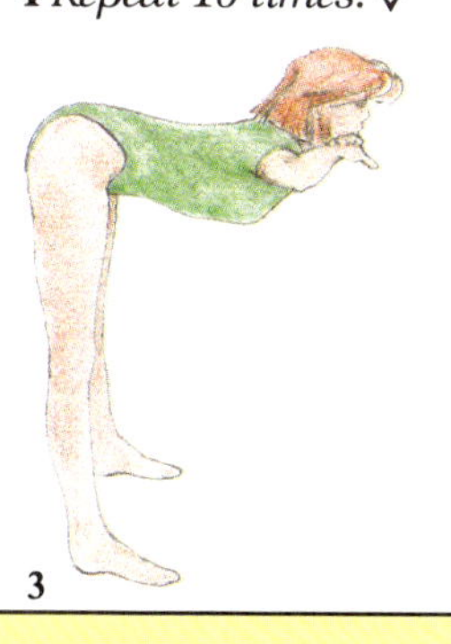

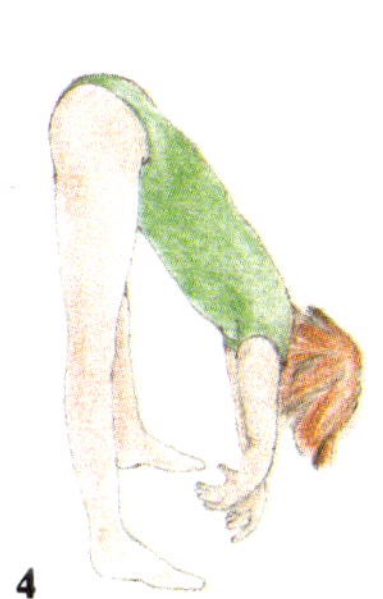

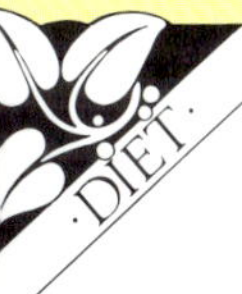

Your vitamin guide — how they affect health and beauty

Throughout the programme it is a good idea for you to supplement your daily diet with vitamin pills. These organic substances are essential for good health and occur naturally in many of the diet foods and recipes. They help protect you against infection, pollution and stress, and have many beauty benefits, too, as they can affect the state of your skin and hair. Stepping up your level of exercise puts your body under greater stress, and daily vitamin supplements will help make you feel better and more energetic.

Fat-soluble vitamins, A, D and E, can be stored in your body for long periods, but water-soluble B and C need to be topped up daily. You can either take a multi-vitamin pill which combines small amounts of all the vitamins or take them separately in slightly larger doses. If you have been feeling low or taking the contraceptive pill, you will probably benefit from taking B-complex or brewers yeast, either in powder or tablet form. Here's a short guide to some of the vitamins and their sources (RDA stands for recommended daily allowance).

Of course, if you eat a really healthy diet all the time, you probably get all the vitamins you need without taking supplements as well. Check the column of natural food sources to ensure that you are eating several foods from each section every day.

Vitamin	Source	Function	RDA
A	Fish liver oils, dairy foods, egg yolks, green vegetables, carrots	Smooth skin, good eyesight	5000iu
B1 Thiamine	Liver, whole grain cereals and bread, nuts, seeds	Good muscle tone, healthy nervous system, stamina	1.0mg
B2 Riboflavin	Meat, liver, fish, eggs, milk, green vegetables	Healthy skin, hair and nails	1.5mg
Niacin	Meat, liver, poultry, fish, whole grain bread, green vegetables, milk, peanuts	Healthy metabolism, good circulation	13mg
B6 Pyridoxine	Meat, liver, fish, brown rice, whole grain bread, banana	Growth, making skin collagen	2.0mg
C	All citrus fruits, blackcurrants, green vegetables, peppers, tomatoes, potatoes	Good skin, healthy teeth and gums, fighting stress	50mg
D	Fish liver oils, tuna, egg yolks, exposure to sunlight	Healthy bones and teeth	400iu
E	Vegetable oils, whole grain cereals, nuts, eggs, avocado	Strong muscles, good circulation	12iu
K	Yoghurt, green vegetables	Liver function and blood clotting	200mcg

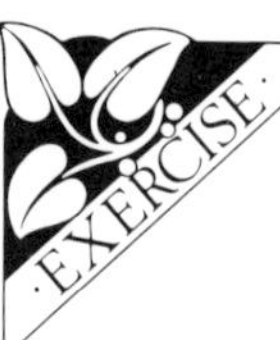

Get off to a running start and slim down your waist

More jogging today, so do your warm-up stretching exercises plus the new ones shown here and then jog/walk as before for 15 minutes. Don't be tempted to overdo it and go too far or too fast — you *must* build up gradually or you may injure yourself. Try to run on soft ground or grass rather than a hard road surface which is more jarring to your back, legs and muscles. But make sure that the ground is not uneven or potholed with tussocks of grass that could make you trip or interfere with the rhythm of your stride. If you are running on the roads after dark or in poor light, wear some white clothing or reflective strips to make you visible in car headlights.

After your run, stretch out your leg muscles again and then relax in a bath. Massage your legs gently to ease out any tension and avoid stiffness. Then it's time to do some waist-trimming exercises. By repeating these exercises every day you can slim down your waist, strengthen back muscles and tone up the whole area.

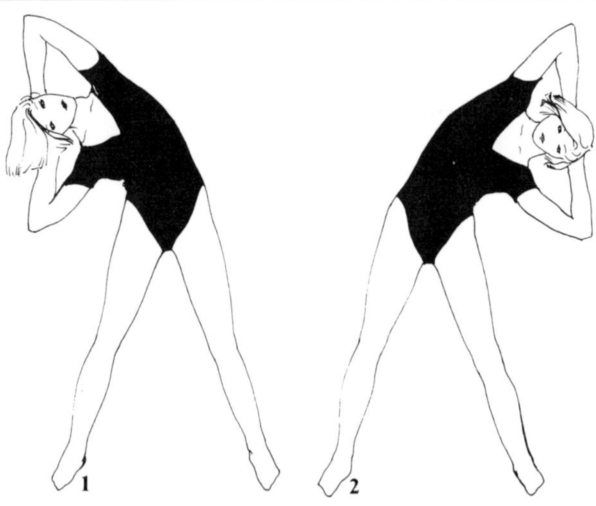

Elbow side stretch
1 *Standing with feet hip distance apart, clasp hands behind head and pull over to right. Repeat 8 times.*
2 *Pull over to the left, keeping feet flat on floor, bending from waist only. Repeat 8 times, alternate from side to side 8 times.*

Trunk lunge
Another running warm-up stretch. Stand with left leg bent in front and right leg outstretched behind. Arch your back and stretch your neck back so that your head is facing upwards. Hold for 20 seconds.

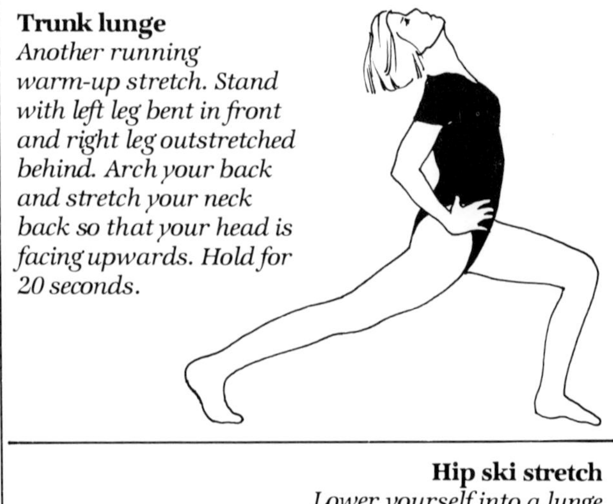

Hip ski stretch
Lower yourself into a lunge position with left leg bent forwards and right leg outstretched behind. Rest on your hands and hold for 20 seconds. Change legs. Repeat.

Twist n'toe touch

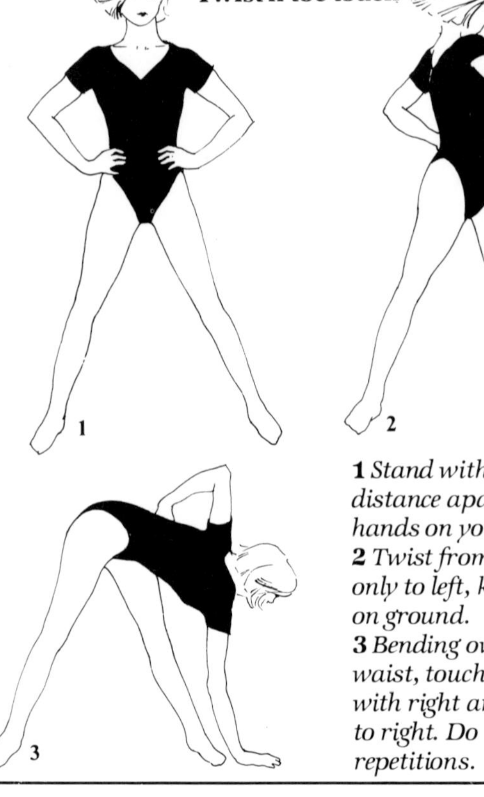

1 *Stand with feet hip distance apart. Rest hands on your waist.*
2 *Twist from waist only to left, keeping feet on ground.*
3 *Bending over from waist, touch left foot with right arm. Repeat to right. Do 10 repetitions.*

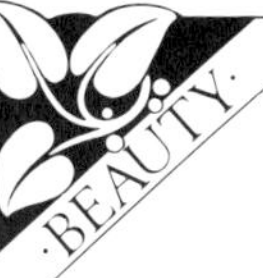

Skin — the bare essentials of keeping in moisture

After being covered up all winter your skin will probably be pale, flaky and tired-looking. If you're going to bare it on the beach, you need to work on it to make it silky and supple. Today's the day to buy some moisturising cream if you don't have some already. You will probably need two different types — one for your face and the other for your body. Before going to bed tonight, moisturise really well. In the morning your skin will look rested, plumped out and fresh. Add some aromatic oil to your bath and moisturise all over with a cooling body lotion. If you don't want a tan to take its toll of you, your skin must be moist and soft to withstand the harmful, drying effects of the sun. So start preparing it now and laying the foundations for a beautiful summer tan later on. Moisturising is a good habit to get into as you will need to do it at least twice daily as part of your after-sun care. It is the key to keeping skin looking young and feeling soft. The older you are, the more important it becomes — from your late twenties onwards you should be very vigilant about moisturising as it can help retard the natural ageing process in your skin.

Modern centrally heated and air-conditioned environments both contribute to dry skin. To ensure that the air is not too dry, why not install a humidifier to replace lost moisture in the atmosphere? They are not expensive and have far-reaching beauty benefits for your skin. As you get older, there is a slowing-down of cell growth and more dead cells on the surface of your skin. Water-in-oil moisturisers will prevent it losing its natural moisture and drying out even further.

Holiday tip

Get your tan off to a good start with a course of sun-bed treatments. Enrol at a local beauty salon or health club and gradually build up a base tan over the next four weeks before you depart for your holiday. Even under a sun-lamp you should still protect your skin with a good sunscreen (see pages 30/31) depending on your degree of vulnerability. If you develop a tan now, you will feel more confident on the beach and can spend more of your precious holiday time enjoying the sun rather than hiding from it in the shade. You will get a deeper tan, too. When you return home afterwards, have another course of treatments to top it up and make it last longer.

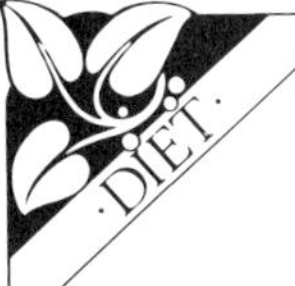

Switch over to mineral water and spring-clean your body

Perhaps you find the idea of buying bottled water shocking or extravagant, but the water that comes out of our taps contains about 1500 pollutants and chemical substances, many of which are cancer-forming and potentially damaging to health in the long run. So forget your scruples and invest in bottled mineral water which is full of natural goodness. A wide range of still and sparkling waters are now on sale in most supermarkets and health food stores. The French ones, which have been scrutinised and graded by the French government, are probably the best and most pure. Drink with ice and a twist of lemon or add a splash of fresh fruit juice — orange or grapefruit.

Of course, not all of the water in your diet comes from what you drink — nearly half your daily water intake comes from food, especially fruit and vegetables. Water is essential for good health and helps spring-clean and detoxify your body. Because it contains no calories, it can be drunk freely without fear of weight gain. Try experimenting with bottled waters — you will be surprised at how different they can taste. Some are pure and still mountain water, others are sparkling or highly mineralised. Remember that spring water and mineral water are not the same thing so opt for the healthy benefits of mineral water.

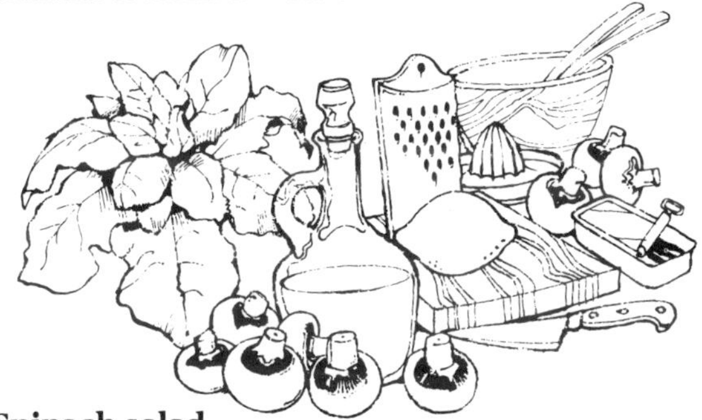

Spinach salad

Handful washed young spinach leaves
50g/2oz button mushrooms, sliced
2 anchovy fillets, chopped
1 spring onion, chopped
15ml/1 tablespoon olive oil
good squeeze lemon juice
5ml/1 teaspoon grated lemon rind

Remove any hard stalks from spinach and place in a bowl with mushrooms, anchovies and onion. Shake up oil and lemon to make a dressing and toss the salad.

Day 4

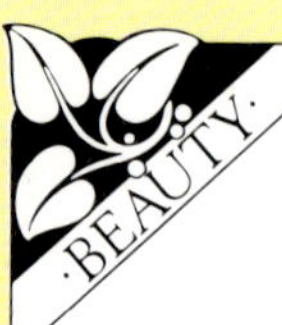

Revive and cleanse your skin with a soothing face mask

A good face mask can cleanse your skin deep down and leave it plump, pink and glowing with health. You can buy a mask or make up your own with natural ingredients from the larder and refrigerator. If you have oily skin, choose a clay, earth or seaweed based mask. Delicate, sensitive skins are better suited to a gentler peel-off mask which hardens to a transparent film across your face, tightening the skin underneath. Make sure you remove any make-up first and then apply according to the manufacturer's instructions, taking care to cover your neck as well as your face. Either peel off or rinse away with water. Repeat the process once every week — twice if your skin is oily.

Or make up your own face mask — try out one of the following suggestions:

1 Mashed avocado and live natural yoghurt. Leave for 20 minutes.

2 Crushed strawberries, a little oatmeal and live yoghurt. Leave for 30 minutes.

3 Beaten egg white with a few drops of lemon juice. Leave for 20 minutes.

For oily skin, try beaten egg yolk with brewers yeast and live natural yoghurt. Dry skins benefit from beaten egg yolk mixed with honey. The enzymes in raw fruit and vegetables are especially good for skin — look at the chart to discover which are best for you. Either use these fruits in face masks or drink their juice daily and you will soon see an improvement in your skin.

Fruit	Skin type	Effects
Apple	Oily, blemished skin	Astringent, antiseptic
Apricot	All skin types	Helps formation of skin cells
Banana	Dry, ageing skin	Moisturising
Cabbage	Blemished skin	Disinfectant, helps heal spots
Carrot	Delicate skin	Heals rashes, moisturises
Cucumber	All skin types	Soothing, bleaching
Grapefruit	Oily, blemished skin	Astringent
Lemon	Oily skin	Astringent, antiseptic
Mint	Oily blemished skin	Soothing, stimulating
Peach	All skin types	Soothing
Strawberry	Oily skin	Toning, astringent

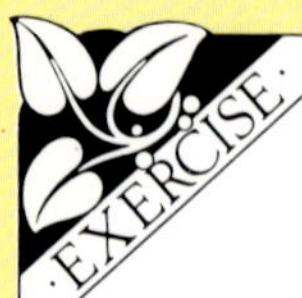

Pedal or plunge into a new exciting aerobic sport

Change your exercise routine today by going for a cycle or visiting your local swimming pool. Both are good forms of aerobic exercise and will burn up calories fast and slim down any fatty deposits.

Cycling: check your bike over before you set out. Make sure that the tyres are pumped up to the right pressure and that brakes are working efficiently. Adjust the height of the seat and handlebars if necessary. Wear loose clothing and set out for a 30 minute cycle. If you get breathless, stop for a short rest before continuing. You should be glowing all over by the time you get home. If you are fairly fit and enjoy cycling, why not cycle to work each day and make it a regular date.

Swimming: if you prefer to pool your efforts, then 30 minutes' swimming will give your body a good work-out. You can use any stroke you wish — breast stroke, crawl or backstroke. It is a good idea to vary strokes as they use different sets of muscles. For example, the breast stroke will tone up hips and the lower back muscles, while the crawl is good for streamlining your body and strengthening shoulder muscles. The back crawl is marvellous for slimming down thighs and working the stomach muscles, whereas sidestroke will trim your waist. Swim as many lengths of the pool as you can, resting when necessary. As you get fitter, you will be able to swim faster and for longer periods without stopping. Choose a time of day when the pool is not too crowded and there are no children to leap in on top of you! Remember to wear a swimming cap to protect your hair from the chlorine in the water. It may also be a good idea to wear goggles as chlorine tends to make your eyes sting. After swimming your skin will probably feel quite dry, so rub in plenty of moisturising cream to keep it soft, smooth and supple.

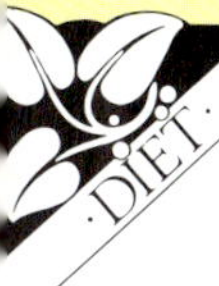

Use aromatic herbs and spices as natural flavourings

We all eat too much salt in our diet, especially hidden salt in many convenience foods. Doctors now believe that a high salt intake is linked with the incidence of heart disease and strokes, so it is a good idea to cut down by using less in cooking and not adding any at the table. Make use of different herbs and exotic spices to add natural flavour to meals. For example, try the following combinations:
Basil with tomatoes and cheese
Chilli with beans
Coriander with aubergines
Dill with salmon
Fennel with fish
Mint with cucumber
Oregano with tomatoes and lettuce
Parsley with fish
Rosemary with courgettes
Sage with chicken and calves liver
Tarragon with chicken
Thyme with potatoes and swedes
For the best results grind the spices yourself in a pestle and mortar, and use really fresh herbs from the garden or your kitchen window box. They will add a new dimension to your cooking and it is fun to experiment with new dishes and flavours. You can also buy a salt substitute at most health food stores if you really are a salty food addict and can't do without it.

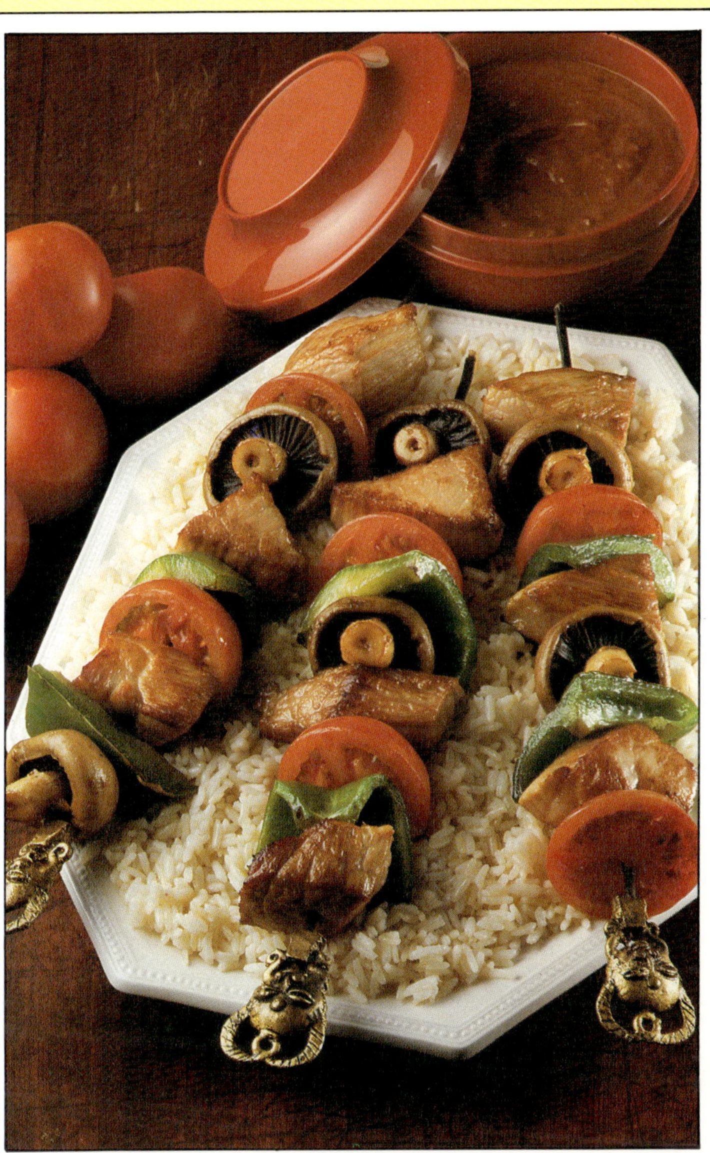

Grilled kebabs

175g/6oz pork fillet or chicken breast
15ml/1 tablespoon oil
good squeeze lemon juice
½ green pepper, cut in chunks
3 cherry tomatoes, halved
5 mushrooms

Cut pork or chicken in large chunks and marinate in oil and lemon for at least 1 hour. Thread onto kebab skewers with the pepper, tomatoes and mushrooms. Brush with any remaining marinade. Grill until cooked right through, turning occasionally. This takes about 12-15 minutes. Serve on a bed of rice (preferably brown) with a fresh green salad or puréed tomatoes.

Holiday tip

If you want your hair to look good on holiday, now is the time to visit the hairdresser and invest in a good cut. Look at different styles in magazines for ideas and ask your hairdresser's advice. Remember, though, that the final decision is yours so don't be cajoled into a style you're unsure about. If you are nervous about cutting off long tresses or having a complete change, then go half-way this time or have a moderated version. You can always make another visit just before you leave if you feel like going the whole way and being adventurous.

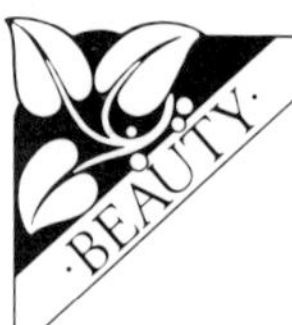

Learn to look after your tell-tale summer nails

Give yourself a home manicure and learn how to get your nails in great shape and tip-top condition. Healthy nails reflect your own good health, and are strong, smooth and pink — not brittled, split or ridged with white spots. Keep your skin soft with a moisturising hand cream, and be sure to wear rubber gloves when washing up, gardening and doing household chores. A weekly manicure is essential to keep nails looking their best, so put aside an hour before you go to bed and get together some emery boards, orange sticks, cotton wool, nail polish remover and a bowl of warm soapy water. You will also need hand cream or cuticle cream.

1 Soak some cotton wool in polish remover and remove any traces of old varnish. Then file the nails into a pretty oval, working inwards from the sides to the centre.
2 Massage nails and fingers with hand cream, nail cream or petroleum jelly. Then soak in warm soapy water for 2-3 minutes. Dry thoroughly.
3 Use an orange stick wrapped around with a little damp cotton wool to ease back the cuticles and then gently rub in some nail cream.
4 Wash your hands. If you are using nail polish, brush evenly with a base hardening coat and then apply a colour coat, brushing upwards from base to tip. Allow to dry and then apply a second coat. A good tip is to brush it just under the tip of each nail to prevent any chipping. When dry, you can apply a protective lacquer, or buff the nails to give them a rosy sheen. Then moisturise your hands. And if your nails break, you can now buy a special kit which repairs them. A thin paper and glue are all that are needed, and the join is disguised by skilfully applied polish over the top.

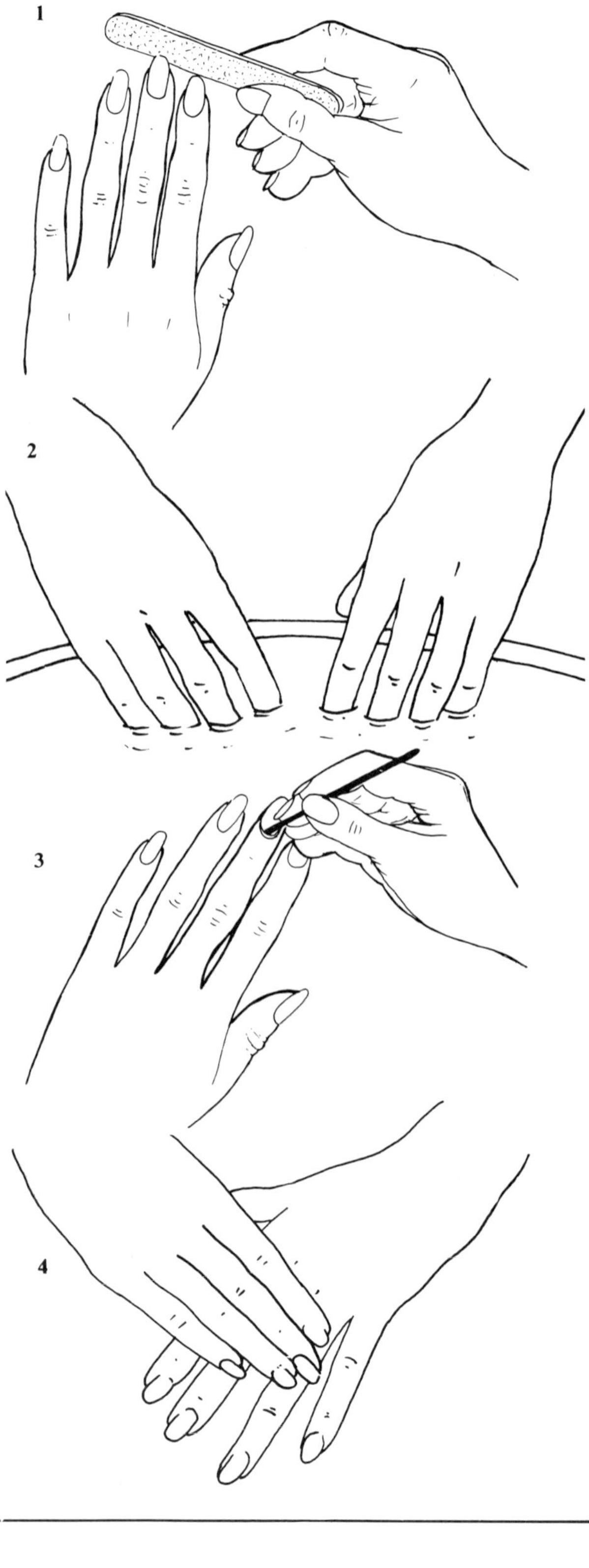

1

2

3

4

Holiday tip

If you are going on a motoring holiday at home or abroad, book your car into a reputable garage for a service before you leave. Make sure that tyres, brakes and lights are thoroughly inspected and any annoying vibrations or noises put right. Also, check your spares kit — spare tyre has proper tread, spanners, jack, tow rope, fan belt, hose, fuses, distributor cap etc. It is also a good idea to keep a first-aid kit in the car together with maps, car compass, torch and fire extinguisher.

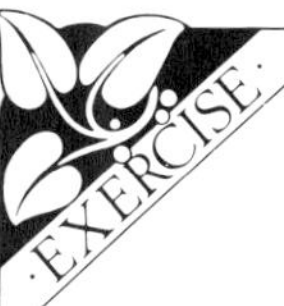

Skip into Day 5 with a new form of aerobic exercise

Let's try a different aerobic exercise today — skipping. This is the cheapest and simplest all-over conditioner and toner of all. Although you may not have skipped since you were very young it is well worth having another go. Practised regularly, skipping will strengthen your leg muscles, build up stamina and burn up calories fast. All you need is a rope and you can do it anywhere — at home, in the garden, in the park or on the beach. It sounds simple and looks easy but, as you will soon find out, it is very hard work indeed.

Start off by skipping for at least three minutes non-stop. You should aim for 70-80 jumps per minute. Repeat three times today, slotting it in around your other activities. Start off with a forwards skip but as you get better, try introducing different steps — backwards and even cross-over skips (see diagrams). Do your leg stretching exercises before you start and then be sure to jump high enough to clear the rope. Look straight ahead — not down at your feet — and breathe evenly and deeply. You will need to wear some running shoes or trainers to cushion the shock as your feet hit the ground with each skip. Build your skipping into the weekly programme so that you skip at least four times a week *in addition* to your other exercises.

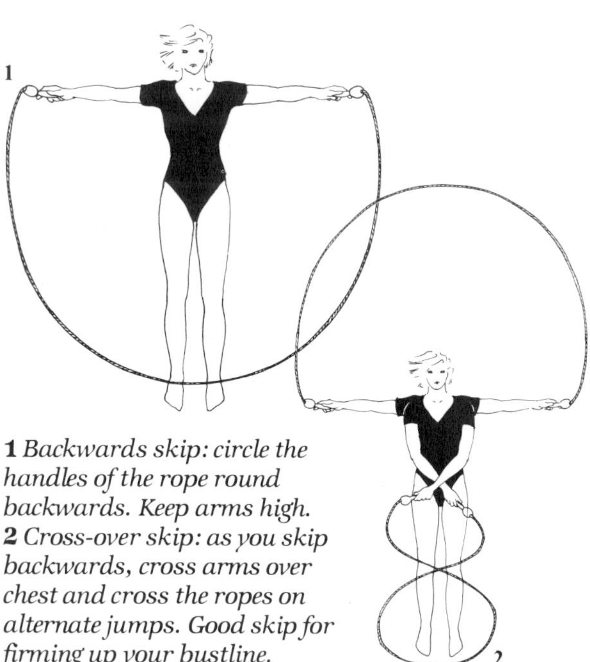

1 *Backwards skip: circle the handles of the rope round backwards. Keep arms high.*
2 *Cross-over skip: as you skip backwards, cross arms over chest and cross the ropes on alternate jumps. Good skip for firming up your bustline.*

Make more time for leisure with labour-saving gadgets

If you have a busy lifestyle — a demanding job and active social life or a family to look after — then you will find it easier if you streamline your cooking and the time spent preparing meals. Good planning and modern electric appliances can help enormously, especially on a healthy eating programme. A blender is a *must* for whizzing up cold summer soups, fruit drinks and vegetable purées. It would take hours to do them by hand. Likewise, a food processor can make fresh wholemeal bread, chop salad vegetables, purée hot and cold soups and generally take the labour out of cooking. A freezer is another boon. Use it for storing your surplus garden vegetables and fruit, extra loaves of bread and even cooked meals that have been prepared in advance. If you haven't much time for shopping, then buy extra fresh fish and poultry and freeze until needed. And if you really are in a hurry, frozen food can be defrosted in seconds in a microwave. Don't be a martyr in the kitchen — make use of all the modern gadgets to ease your workload and create more time for other things. A quickly prepared dinner is over sooner, allowing you more time to go for a walk or attack the beauty programme. Don't scorn modern technology — make it work for you!

Gazpacho

1 large tomato, skinned
¼ green pepper, seeded and diced
large chunk cucumber, chopped
½ stick celery, chopped
1 clove garlic, crushed
2 spring onions, chopped
juice of ½ lemon
sprig parsley
dash of Tabasco
salt and pepper
75ml/3floz tomato juice

Blend all the ingredients together. Chill well and serve with ice cubes. Ideal soup for a hot day.

Day 6

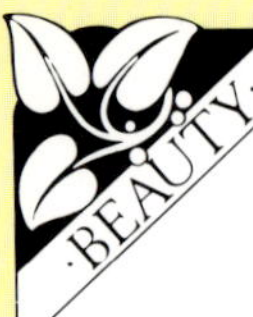

Treat your hair to a deep conditioning treatment

Time to give your hair a deep conditioning treatment, especially if it is dry or brittle with split ends. This is quite different from the conditioner you apply after shampooing. It works deeply on your hair and scalp to leave hair glossy and soft. And it will make tinted or permed hair more manageable and resilient. Most conditioners of this kind need to be left on the hair for 15-20 minutes if they are to be effective. If your hair is damaged, repeat the exercise every week, but once a month should be sufficient for normal hair. You can buy a hot wax or oil conditioner or you can make your own.
If your hair is very dry: shampoo and rinse in the normal way until really clean. Towel-dry. Now massage about 45ml/3 tablespoons of warm olive oil mixed with a little hot water into your scalp. Rub it in well and then wrap your head in a hot wet towel. Leave for 20 minutes before rinsing thoroughly. Shampoo again and finish off with a normal conditioning cream rinse. Style and dry. Really dry damaged hair will get even worse if it is not put right before you get to the sun, the sea and chlorinated swimming pools. Use a pH-balanced protein pack and conditioner twice weekly until the condition improves, and be careful not to use an over-hot hairdryer, heated rollers and curling tongs. Nor should you over-brush hair with a sharp-bristled brush.
If your hair is normal or oily: shampoo and rinse well. Towel-dry. Rub a mixture of beaten egg and a little olive oil and cider vinegar into your hair and scalp. Roll a hot damp towel around your head and leave for 20 minutes. Rinse, shampoo again and then use a cream conditioner. Rinse, set and dry. After one of these treatments, your hair should look really glossy and silky. Another good tip for oily hair is to add the freshly squeezed juice of a whole lemon to the final rinse. The astringent juice will help control excess oil and close up over-active follicles.

If you have ever wondered how a conditioner works here's the explanation: it coats each hair with a fine protective film, usually of balsam or protein, which adds strength and thickness, smoothes down the cuticle and keeps in its natural moisture.

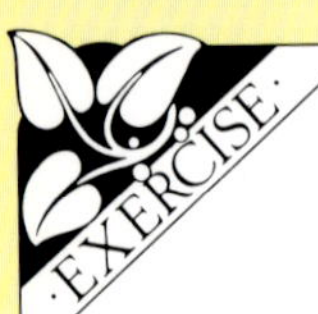

Run for fun and work on beating a bulging tummy

Make time for a short run today. Follow your usual routine — stretch, run/walk for 15 minutes, stretch again and shower. Here are some exercises for strengthening your stomach muscles. Whether you have a spare tyre or not, you should have a go at these abdominal exercises as they will help trim and firm up your middle, get rid of nasty bulges and improve muscle tone. You will not only be fitter and slimmer but this sort of exercise will help improve your overall endurance so that you can run, cycle and swim better and more easily.

To test your abdominal fitness, see how many sit-ups you can do comfortably in one minute. Sit on the floor with knees bent and feet anchored under a chair or bed (or get a friend to hold them down on the floor). Put your hands behind your head and lean forwards so that your chin touches your knees. Now lean back but don't touch down on the ground; come up again and touch your knees with your chin. You should feel your stomach muscles working hard. Keep doing these sit-ups for 60 seconds and see how many you can do.

Level of fitness	No. of sit-ups
Poor to average	5 - 15
Quite fit	16 - 29
Very fit	over 30

Improve your abdominal muscles by repeating these sit-ups every day, gradually increasing the number as you get fitter. Try these other exercises, too.

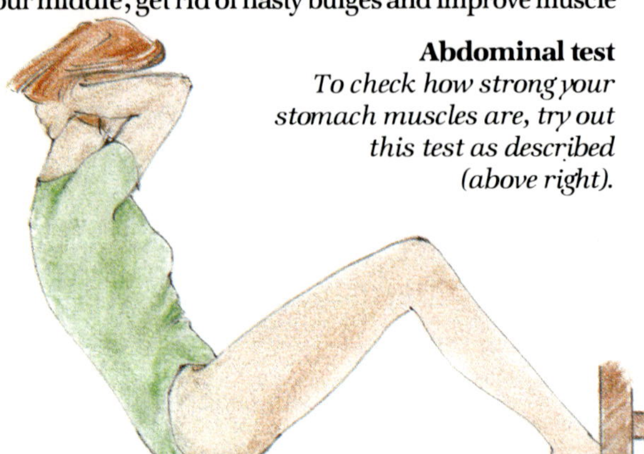

Abdominal test
To check how strong your stomach muscles are, try out this test as described (above right).

Bicycle ▷
1 *Lie with hands behind head. Bend right knee to left elbow, feet flexed.*
2 *Reverse feet and repeat 15 times. Then repeat another 15 times with toes pointed.*

Keep unwanted extra weight at bay with exercise

Did you know that too much dieting can make you fat? This may sound ridiculous but many doctors and nutritional experts believe it to be true. It seems that strict reducing diets slow down the body's metabolic rate so that although some fluid is lost, the fat is burned up more slowly. In fact, if you don't exercise, you are more likely to lose lean tissue and muscle than fat as your body adapts to having less food and its functions slow down. However, by exercising regularly you are more likely to lose fat than muscle. This is because your body needs it for physical activity and so it sheds the unwanted fat. Exercise can speed up metabolic rate and burn foods more quickly. It can curb hunger pangs and is the only way to keep weight permanently at bay and avoid the vicious circle of over-eating and dieting. By sticking to your programme of diet and exercise every day, you can be confident that you are losing body fat and increasing your proportion of lean tissue. Thus even though you may be over-fat, you may not be overweight. Exercise can convert, say, 3kg/7lb of fat into lean tissue, so that although you weigh the same your body shape changes and you look slimmer with well-toned-up muscles.

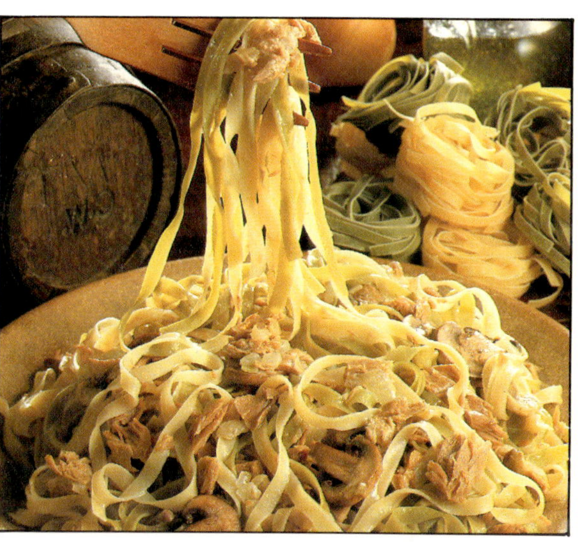

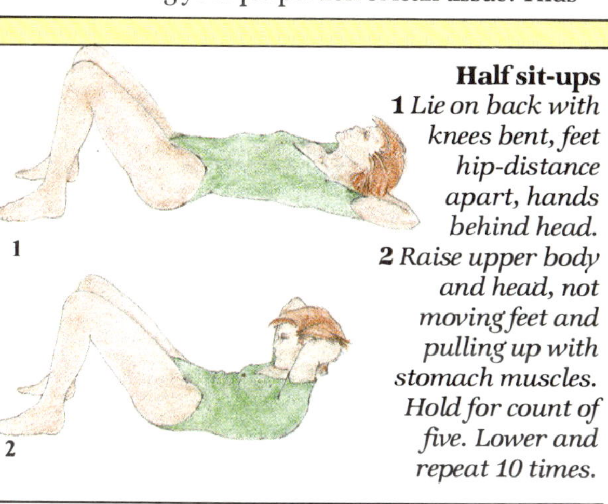

Half sit-ups

1 *Lie on back with knees bent, feet hip-distance apart, hands behind head.*

2 *Raise upper body and head, not moving feet and pulling up with stomach muscles. Hold for count of five. Lower and repeat 10 times.*

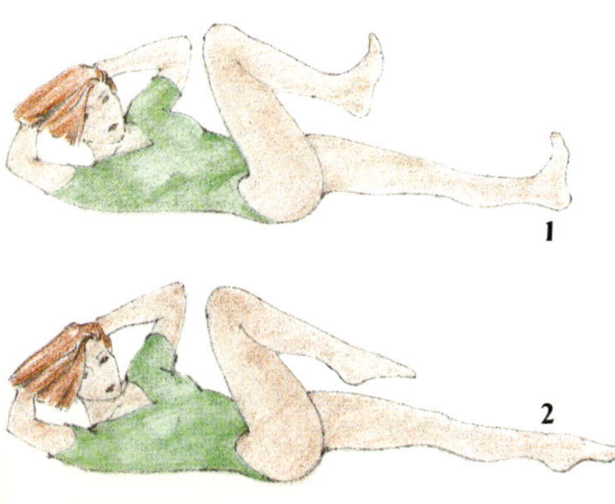

Tagliatelle al tonno

75g/3oz tagliatelle
½ onion, chopped
50g/2oz mushrooms, sliced
salt and black pepper
50g/2oz canned tuna fish
50ml/2floz natural yoghurt

Cook tagliatelle until tender. Drain and keep warm. Sauté onion in a little oil until soft. Add mushrooms and seasoning. Cook 3 minutes. Add tuna and tagliatelle. Stir in yoghurt and heat through gently to avoid curdling.

Holiday tip

Why not have a weekly sauna to cleanse your system and clear out waste and pollutants? It helps attack cellulite (see page 28) and is a great beauty treatment for your skin, cleansing it deep down. Most health clubs and many sports and recreation centres have sauna baths, and they are not usually expensive. After your sauna, lie down for 30 minutes and rest while you let your body readjust to a lower temperature. Don't expect great weight loss — any fluid you lose in the sauna will soon be replaced when you have a drink and a meal. If you get the opportunity, have a massage afterwards to further stimulate circulation and soothe tense muscles.

Day 7

Wage war on cellulite with diet, friction and massage

Check your hips and thighs for cellulite — the puffy, dimpled fat which affects only women and looks rather puckered like orange skin. It is sometimes also found on the shoulders, upper arms, stomach, ankles and buttocks. Bad diet, a build-up of waste matter and pollutants in the body and a lack of exercise all contribute to the condition. Sticking to your new healthy diet will help prevent future cellulite forming. Be sure to avoid over-processed foods like sugar, bacon, sausages, processed ham and cheese, smoked and pickled products, salted nuts and crisps. Alcohol is another hazard as are caffeine drinks such as tea and coffee.

Make sure you drink plenty of mineral water to flush out your system, and at least three glasses of vegetable juice daily — beetroot, carrot, celery, cucumber or watercress — to remove any toxic wastes. Keep this up throughout the programme. Cucumber is especially beneficial as it is diuretic and firms up soggy tissues. Although spring-cleaning from within your body helps a great deal, you have to tackle cellulite on the outside, too. Friction and massage are both effective treatments. They physically break down the cellulite pockets, improve circulation in these deadened areas and help step up metabolism of the cells and eliminate any wastes. Here's how to do it:

1 In the bath or shower, attack any patches of cellulite with a massage glove which holds a bar of specially formulated soap, or use a rough massage mit to boost circulation, remove any dead skin cells and vibrate the skin. You can put a handful of coarse table salt on the mit to exfoliate it thoroughly.

2 Massage some anti-cellulite cream into the skin. The ones based on ivy, seaweed and horse-chestnut are all good. Do it after your bath when the skin is warm and receptive with open pores. Stroke it gently at first, hand over hand, stroking away from the heart and increasing the pressure gradually. Now start kneading to draw away any wastes and boost circulation further.

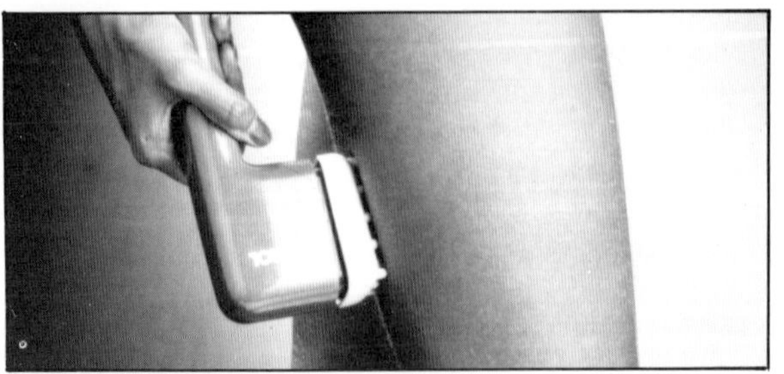

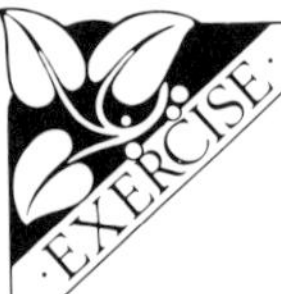

Concentrate today on working your hips and thighs

Work-out to your home exercise tape or at a keep-fit class *or* do all the stretching and work-out exercises you have learnt on the programme to date *plus* these exercises for hips and thighs. These can be problem areas even for slim people and need regular, preferably daily, exercise to break down fatty deposits and tone up sagging muscles. You need strong hips and legs to prevent you tiring at other sports, especially running. If you think you have strong thighs, then try the following test. It sounds easy but you may be surprised at how difficult it is to hold the position for very long. If you are a good skiier you should have no difficulty as your quadriceps muscles will be well-developed. Stand against a wall and, keeping your back straight, slide down the wall into a seated position with your thighs parallel to the ground. Now hold the position for as long as possible. If you are moderately fit, you should be able to sustain it for 20-40 seconds. If your quads are really strong, you can hold it for a minute or more.

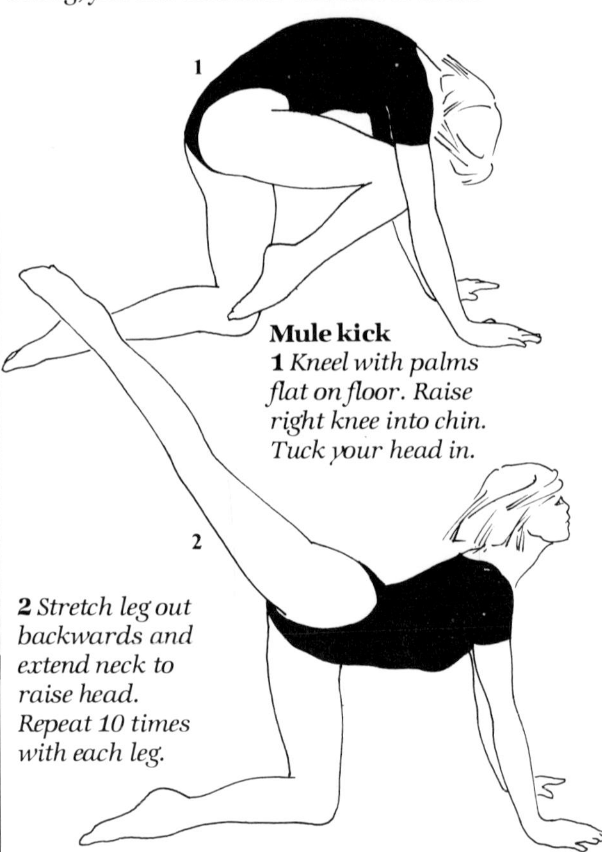

Mule kick
1 *Kneel with palms flat on floor. Raise right knee into chin. Tuck your head in.*

2 *Stretch leg out backwards and extend neck to raise head. Repeat 10 times with each leg.*

Side leg kick

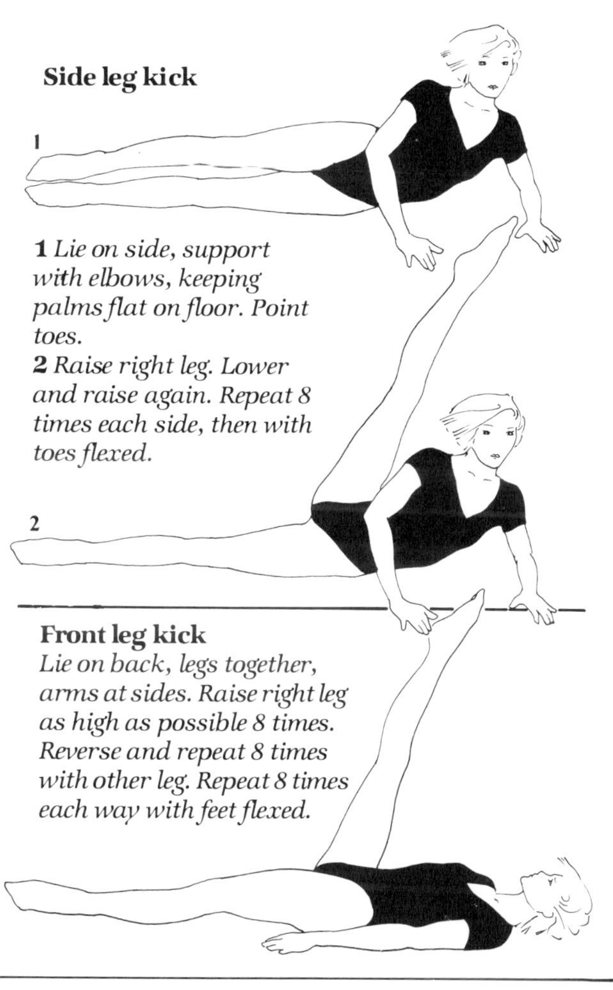

1 *Lie on side, support with elbows, keeping palms flat on floor. Point toes.*
2 *Raise right leg. Lower and raise again. Repeat 8 times each side, then with toes flexed.*

Front leg kick

Lie on back, legs together, arms at sides. Raise right leg as high as possible 8 times. Reverse and repeat 8 times with other leg. Repeat 8 times each way with feet flexed.

Holiday tip

Make sure that you have adequate travel and medical insurance cover for your holiday. Most tour operators offer it when you make your booking although you can make your own arrangements if you prefer. Travel insurance can cover cancellation, luggage, loss of money, personal accident and liability. Check the policy to find out your exact cover. You may also wish to take out medical insurance. If you are a citizen of an EEC country you can take advantage of the reciprocal arrangements which exist. Ask at the appropriate government office for details and forms. If you are travelling outside the EEC, you will need private insurance, especially in the United States where medical expenses can be high. Insurance costs surprisingly little and is well worth it in case of accident, illness or loss, so don't think that you can do without it. You might need it.

Feed your skin from the inside with high-quality food

Your skin reflects your inner state of health and its greatest enemies are stress and poor diet. Many problem skins — oily, blemished, coarse or sallow — are related to processed foods, too much sugar and fat and not enough fresh fruit and vegetables. Changing your diet along the lines laid down in the programme is bound to improve the condition of your skin. It needs high-nutrient food to nourish it, keep it smooth and elastic, soft and blemish-free.

Plenty of high-fibre foods and mineral water will help flush out waste products, whereas vitamin C (citrus fruit, tomatoes, peppers, potatoes, green vegetables, bean sprouts) protects the collagen fibres in your skin and helps prevent wrinkling. Vitamin A (found in carrots, yellow fruits and vegetables, peppers, beans, eggs) helps to keep skin moist and prevent dryness. The B-complex vitamins (whole grain bread and cereals, beans and brewers yeast) aid good circulation and keep skin healthy. Protein is very important, too, for making healthy collagen (the supportive fibres in your skin).

If you have a particular skin problem, you may find it useful to take a vitamin supplement for a while. For example, many people swear by vitamin E as a miracle cure for ageing skin. It is good to take on holiday as it combats the toxic 'free radicals' in the skin formed by the sun's radiation. Just take 200-400ius per day to be on the safe side.

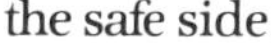

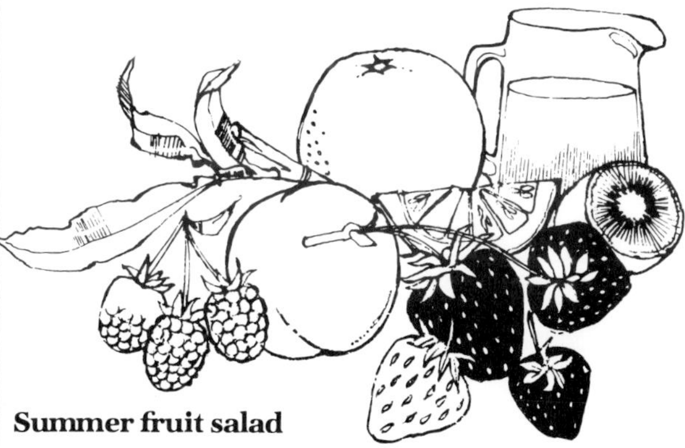

Summer fruit salad

1 orange, segmented
1 peach/nectarine, sliced
few strawberries/raspberries, hulled
½ kiwi fruit, sliced
50-75ml/2-3floz unsweetened orange juice

Prepare the fresh fruit and place in a dish, pour over the orange juice and serve with natural yoghurt if wished.

Holiday suncare

You can judge a good holiday by your tan. Summer bronzed skin is flattering and healthy-looking but it is also your skin's way of protecting itself against the sun's burning rays. You need not suffer the misery of redness and blisters if you prepare your skin before you leave.

Groundwork

Throughout the month leading up to your departure, moisturise your skin every day — not just your face but all over. Use bath oil to keep your skin moist and smooth, and rub away any dead skin cells on the surface with a massage mit or loofah. After bathing or showering, gently rub in a good body lotion.

If the weather is warm and sunny you can get a good foundation tan on which to build later by gradually exposing your skin and building up the time spent sunbathing. Otherwise you might consider a course of sunbed treatments. Inquire about their availability and cost at your local beauty salon or health club. Or you can use an artificial tanning cream or tablets which stain your skin so that you look tanned. But however bronzed you may appear, they cannot offer you protection against the sun and so you will still need to use a strong sunscreen, even though you won't look a paleface on the beach.

How you tan

When you go in the sun, you expose your skin to burning and tanning ultra-violet (UV) rays. Deep down in your skin are melanin granules which contain a dark pigment. These travel to the surface to protect it against sun damage and make your skin look brown and tanned. When you use a sunscreen, it helps block out the burning UV rays so that the tanning UV rays can promote your tan painlessly. People with dark skins have larger, more numerous melanin granules than their fair-skinned sisters and thus they tan more easily.

Your sun protection factor rating

Choosing the right suncare product is very important if you are to reap the rewards of a beautiful golden tan. And there is hope for you even if you have fair, delicate skin. You can still avoid the misery of sunburn and need not suffer in your quest for a tan. Most sunscreen products are graded with a sun protection factor (SPF) number on a scale descending from 15-2. In order to find out which number is best for you, you must first assess your skin type:

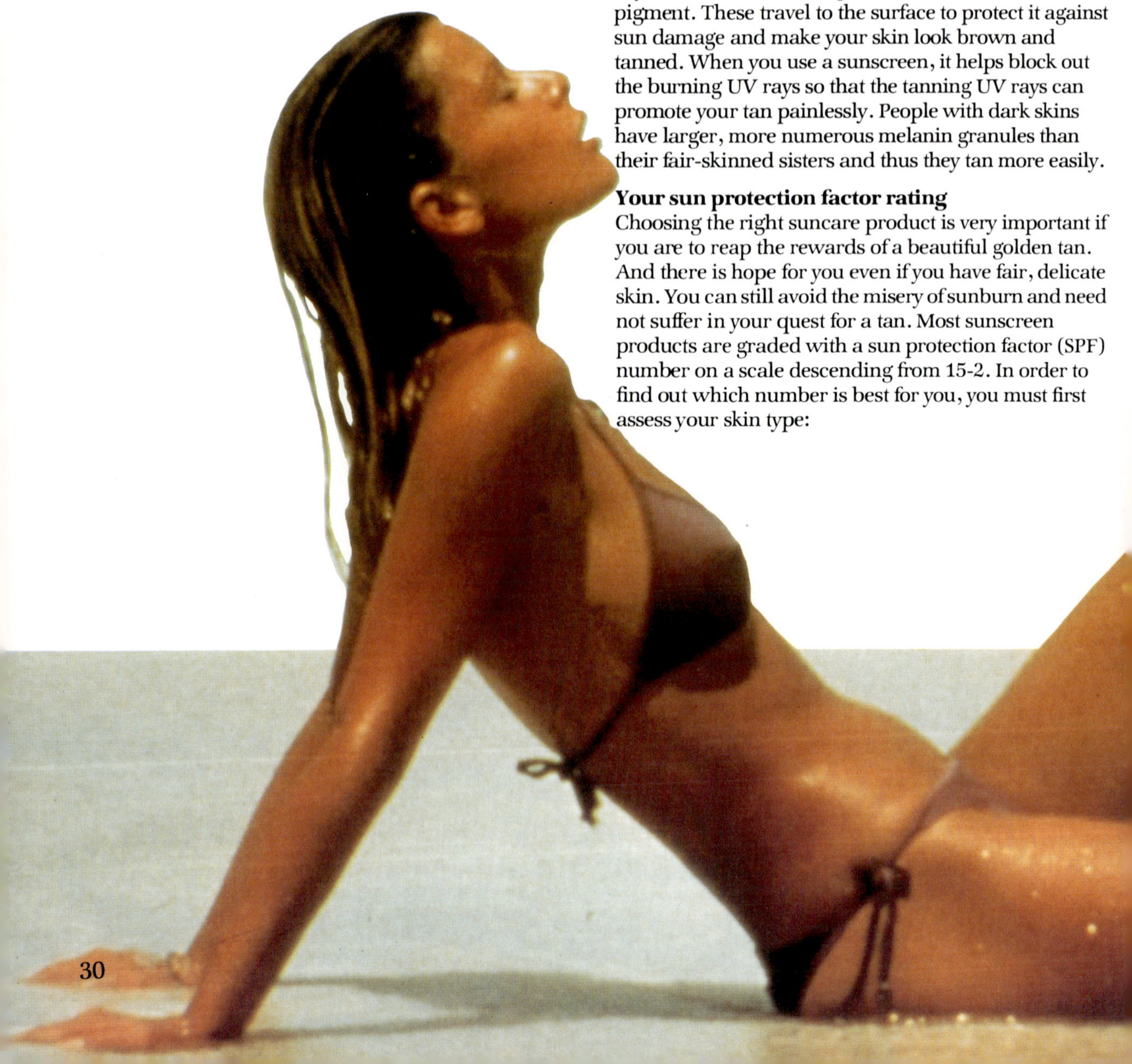

Numbers 15-8 : ideal for pale, sensitive skins which are inclined to burn easily. Start off with a high number and work your way down as your tan progresses.
Numbers 7-5 : good for normal balanced skin types which tan gradually but still need a degree of protection against the sun.
Numbers 4-2 : for lucky people who tan easily and rarely burn, especially olive and dark complexions. But even if you fall into this category you still need some protection and must be sure to use after-sun moisturisers to prevent flaking. You may find that you need to use different numbered sunscreens simultaneously — for example a higher SPF number on your face and vulnerable areas like breasts and stomach than on your arms and legs.

When you arrive...
On your first day on the beach, generously apply the suncream about half an hour before you venture out into the sun — creams and lotions are less effective on wet or perspiring skin. Rub it in gently and uniformly to promote an even tan. Use a high SPF number for maximum protection, but as the days go by and your tan deepens you can gradually descend to a lower number.

Tanning tips
1 When using sun cream don't forget to treat areas like your feet, elbows, backs of knees, breasts, nose and shoulder blades which are very vulnerable.
2 Avoid the really hot midday sun when the burning UV rays are at their strongest. Start off by sunbathing early in the morning and the late afternoon. Relax in the shade around noon with a cool drink, preferably iced fruit juice or mineral water.
3 You can't hide from the sun in the sea. The powerful UV rays penetrate water and can still burn you. Use a special waterproof sunblock for added protection when swimming and reapply afterwards.
4 Even on a hazy or cloudy day you may still be at risk. Although some of the sun's radiation is filtered by light cloud cover, the UV rays are as intense as ever so continue wearing your sunscreen.
5 Always apply a lipscreen regularly to avoid burnt, lips. They contain no oil glands or protective melanin.
6 Limit the amount of time you spend in the sun — not more than about one hour on your first day in a hot climate. Depending on your skin type and sensitivity, you can gradually extend your bouts of bathing.
7 Even when you have a tan, continue using a sunscreen. Although tanned skin affords some protection it cannot block out radiation altogether.

Keeping your tan
If you want to stay tanned after you return home you must moisturise your skin every day to prevent it drying and flaking. Your tan will fade as your skin sheds its outer layers and renews itself from below. When bathing use less soap and pat gently dry instead of rubbing vigorously. Apply a good moisturising body lotion.

If you burn...
Use a soothing medicated lotion or cream, especially one that contains aloe oil, and stay out of the sun or cover any burnt skin until the soreness and redness disappear. Calamine or a mixture of equal parts bicarbonate of soda and water will help take the burn out of sore skin. Taking multi-vitamin tablets and zinc can also help. But you *can* avoid all this pain and discomfort if you take precautions, however delicate or vulnerable your skin may be.

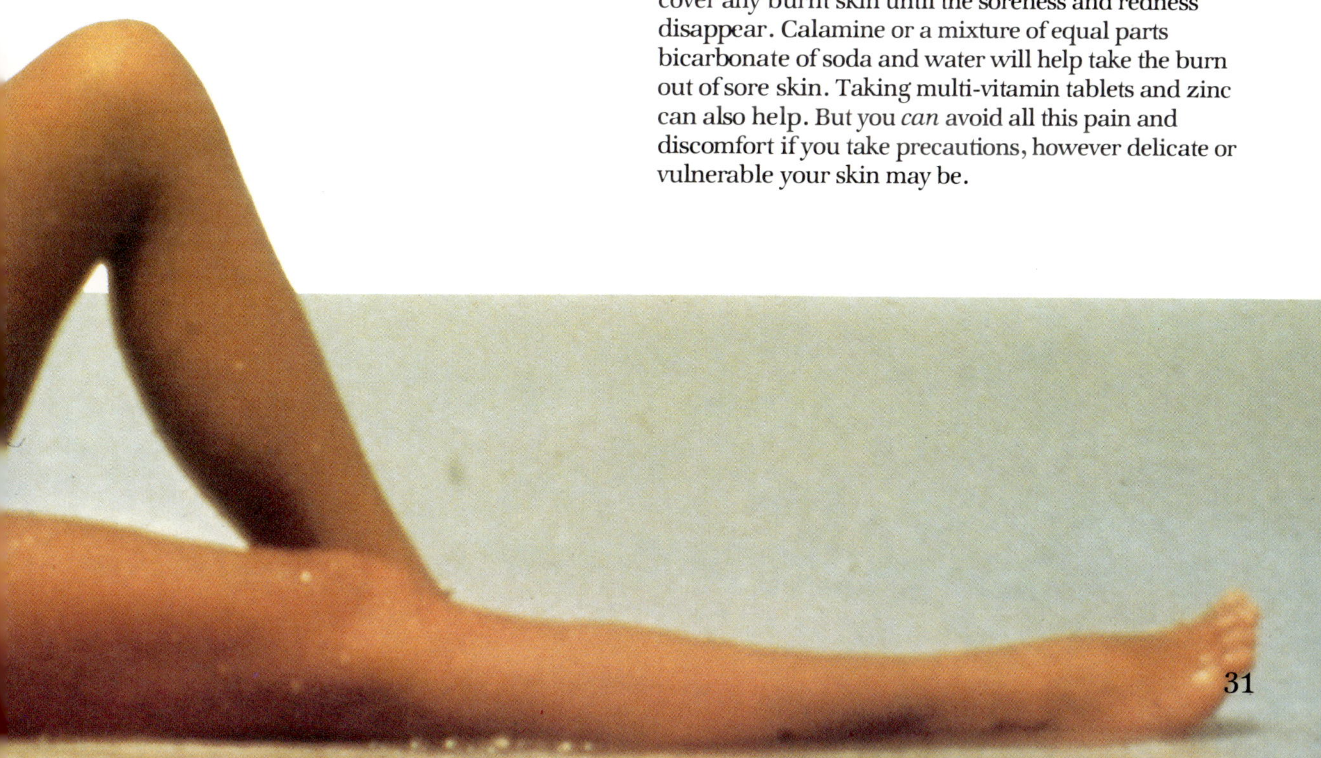

Learn the art of self-massage to stimulate circulation

You do not have to visit a health farm or beauty salon for a good massage. You can have one just as easily at home, either self-administered or in the hands of a friend. All you need is some pure vegetable oil or talcum powder to enable your hands to slide and move more easily across your skin. Safflower, sunflower and olive oil are all acceptable. The best time to have a massage is immediately after a warm bath when your skin is at its most receptive.

The purpose of massage is to relieve muscular tension, stimulate blood flow and to have a gentle tranquillising effect upon your system. It can also be useful in getting rid of cellulite, of course. There are three techniques you need to learn — kneading, friction and stroking (or effleurage). They all break down adhesions and improve circulation. They are also useful in the event of athletic injuries and strains as they help relieve pain. Gently stroking the surface of the skin sedates nerve endings — that's why you learnt to 'rub it better' when you hurt yourself as a child.

Undress and lie down on a mat or blanket on the floor in a warm room. Cover the parts of your body which are not being massaged with a rug. Now move your hands firmly and rhythmically across the skin as described below. Remember that massage should be an enjoyable, not a painful, experience and there is no need to pummel your body into submission!

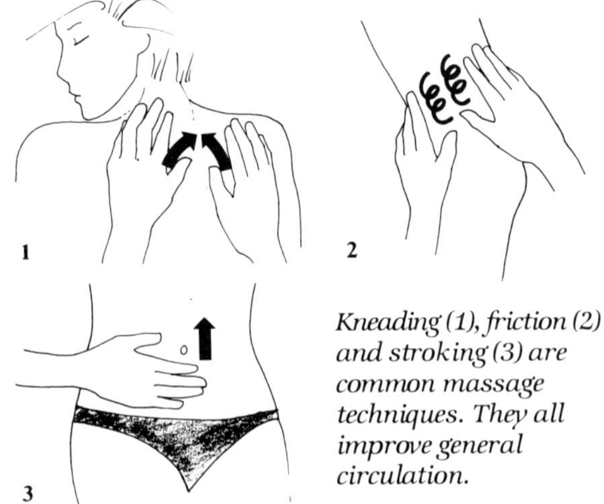

Kneading (1), friction (2) and stroking (3) are common massage techniques. They all improve general circulation.

1 Lie on your back and stroke gently but firmly upwards from your abdomen towards your ribs.
2 As you get more accustomed to the rhythm, press a little harder on each upwards stroke. Then sit up and knead each arm and shoulder gently, paying particular attention to the back of your neck to ease out any tension across the shoulder blades.
3 Massage the backs of your legs, working in strong circular movements and using your knuckles and thumbs to twist and knead any patches of cellulite on hips and thighs.
4 Gradually reduce the pressure and ease down into a firm stroking movement again on your calf muscles (lower legs).
5 Relax — breathe evenly and deeply.

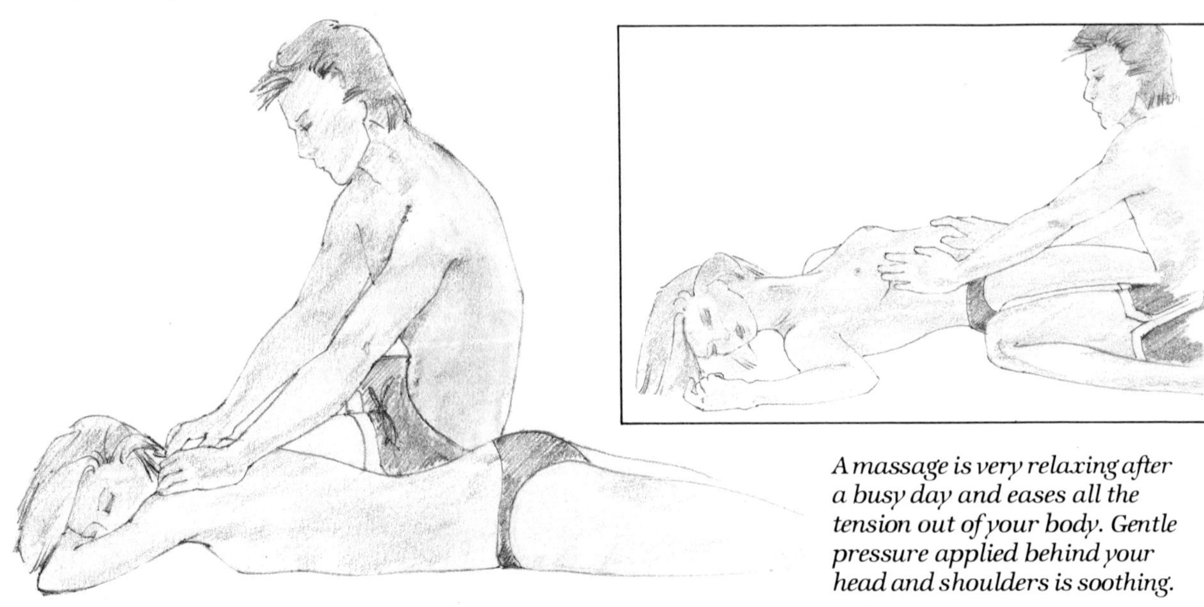

A massage is very relaxing after a busy day and eases all the tension out of your body. Gentle pressure applied behind your head and shoulders is soothing.

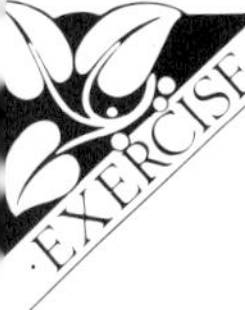

Choose from swimming, cycling or skipping for some great aerobic exercise

You have the choice today of getting out on your bike, twirling a skipping rope or plunging into the swimming pool. Whichever you opt for, try to improve on your performance last time, although be sure not to overdo it or you could end up with sore, aching muscles which will disrupt your exercise programme for a few days.
Skipping: be a bit more adventurous with your skipping today and in addition to your usual routine, try out a new skipping two-step. You will soon master this with a little practice. Begin by jumping over the rope with your knees together. Then, as you get into the rhythm, raise one leg and hop over the rope with the other foot. Repeat 10 times and then swap legs. Keep doing this with alternate legs for as long as you can — aim for at least three minutes. Build this into your regular skipping routine.
Cycling: no fancy acrobatic stunts on your bike but try to cycle a little faster and further than you did last time. Your leg muscles will probably be feeling stronger now and you will have more energy and stamina to push yourself up the hills.
Swimming: warm-up with a few of the stretches you have learnt and then swim a couple of lengths practising your strokes. Now swim for 15 minutes, alternating between two strokes and pushing yourself a little harder.

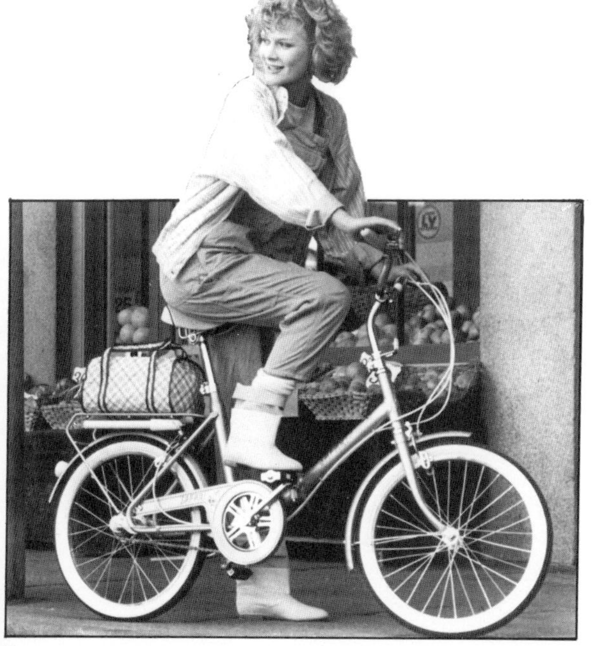

Feed your hair with vitamins and minerals to give it shine and bounce

The food you eat affects the health of your hair just like any other part of your body. If you want your hair to be strong, thick and glossy, you must eat a really healthy diet which contains plenty of vitamins and minerals. Your diet programme is perfect for this as it is highly nutritious and emphasises fresh whole food. Crash slimming diets and too many processed foods, white sugar and refined carbohydrates all cause damage to your hair and upset the delicate balance of nutrients in your body.

The B-complex vitamins are particularly important for keeping hair beautiful and healthy. Taking brewers yeast and vitamin B12 daily will help protect your hair from dandruff, scaling and dullness. Make sure you eat plenty of wholemeal bread, brown rice and green vegetables or take daily supplements. Zinc, sulphur and iron are essential for keeping your hair looking good. Anaemia is a common condition in women which is usually linked to too little iron in the bloodstream. Brittle, split, dull-looking hair which lacks lustre and tends to fall out is often a symptom of anaemia. Visit your doctor if you fear that you might be anaemic. He will probably prescribe a course of iron tablets for you. And eat plenty of liver, green vegetables, spinach, seafoods and whole grains. The iron is absorbed more efficiently when you eat vitamin C as well, so make sure you have some citrus fruit or juice, tomatoes, peppers and green vegetables as well.

Rice stuffed pepper

1 large red or green pepper
50g/2oz brown rice
½ small onion, chopped
5ml/1 teaspoon oil
50g/2oz diced feta cheese or cooked chicken
1 tomato, skinned and chopped
chopped fresh herbs
salt and pepper
5ml/1 teaspoon grated Parmesan cheese

Slice the top stalk end off pepper and scoop out seeds. Cook brown rice in boiling water until tender and drain. Sauté onion in oil and mix into cooked rice with cheese/chicken, tomato, herbs and seasoning. Stuff pepper and sprinkle with Parmesan cheese. Stand in baking tray filled with a little water and bake at 180°C/350°/gas 4 for about 1 hour.

Day 9

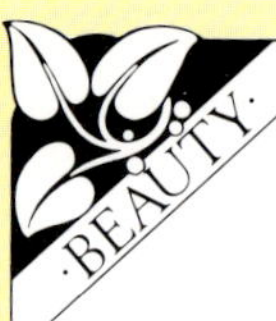

Be a bathing beauty and enjoy a relaxing bath after a busy day

A warm bath is soothing and refreshing at the end of a hard day. Have one tonight last thing before going to bed. For a warm, luxurious wallow, the temperature should be between 29°-34°C/85°-95°F. Add some perfumed bath oil to the water to make your skin moist and sweet-smelling. Natural oils, available from most health shops, are best. Choose one of the following:

- Lime and lavender are relaxing and encourage sleep
- Walnut oil for problem skin
- Pine and thyme are invigorating

Other fragrant oils include rosemary, citron, patchouli, jasmine and rose. All you need are a few drops and, unlike most bath foams and detergent-based products, they will not dry or irritate your skin.

Before you bathe, rub yourself vigorouslly all over with some coarse sea salt to remove any dead skin cells and encourage circulation. In the bath, don't just lie there — do the exercises shown and use a loofah on rough knees and elbows. Attack the soles of your feet with a pumice stone. Afterwards, vigorously rub yourself dry with a towel to create friction and slough off dead cells. Then gently massage your skin with a moisturising oil or body lotion. It will feel soft and silky. Make this part of your regular routine, or do it at least twice a week. It will help prepare your skin for holiday sunshine. The softer and better moisturised it is, the more it will be able to withstand the drying effects of salt-water, sea breezes, swimming pools and ultra-violet rays.

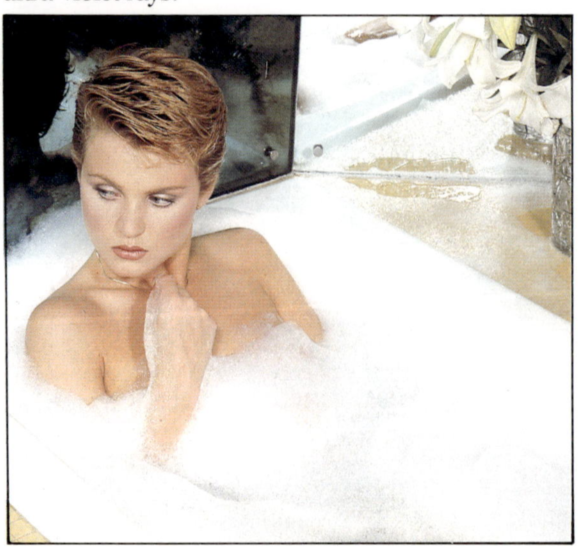

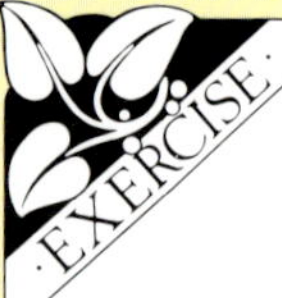

Lengthen your jogging distance and have a bathing work-out

Jogging again today, so follow the now-familiar pattern of stretch, jog/walk for 15 minutes, then stretch and relax in a bath. If you can now run for 15 minutes non-stop, think about increasing it to 20 minutes next time you go out. However, don't worry if you haven't yet surmounted this hurdle. Take your time and build up gradually — you are probably feeling fitter and stronger already and can run a little further and faster than you did when you started out last week.

In the bath, try out some exercises. They will help firm and tone up muscles, especially abdominals and legs. Use a bath mat to stop you sliding about. Start off with some alternate leg kicks, 20 times with each leg, taking care not to splash too much water around the bathroom! Now, holding the sponge between your feet, raise your legs slowly and hold for a count of five. Slowly lower and then raise again. Repeat 10 times. Now carry on with the exercises shown.

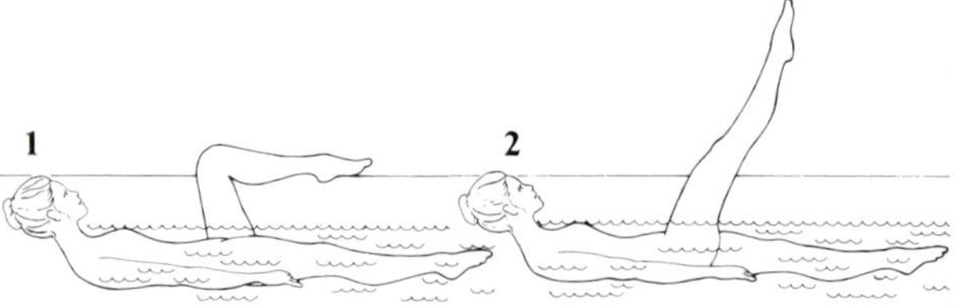

Leg kicks

1 *Lie back in the bath, head raised and arms at your sides. Bend one leg above the water level.*

2 *Extend the leg as high as it will go with pointed toes. Lower and repeat 15 times with both legs.*

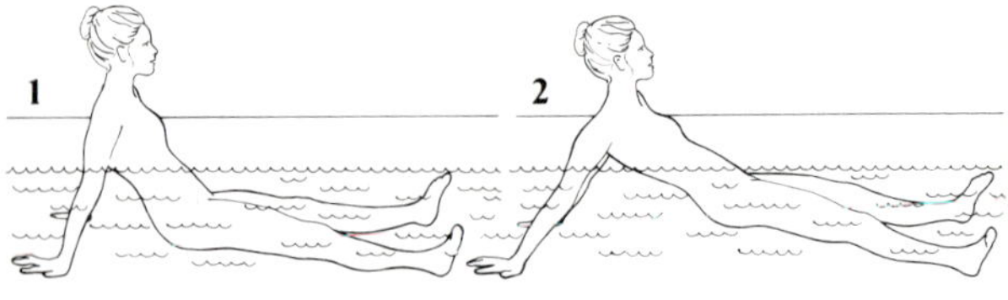

Stomach tightener

1 *Sit in bath with legs a little apart and stomach pulled in. Support yourself with your arms.*

2 *Use stomach muscles to raise bottom slightly while sliding arms backwards. Slowly pull yourself up to starting position. Repeat 10 times.*

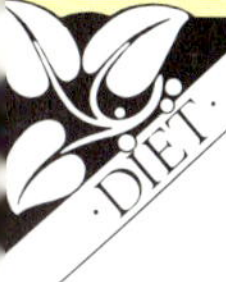

Discover the full of fitness foods for lasting energy

Natural whole foods are ideal for keeping your body healthy and energetic. Athletes in training for a marathon tend to eat lots of high-quality foods, especially raw fibre-rich fruit, vegetable salads, nuts, seeds and whole grains. You do not have to eat extra protein to make you stronger, contrary to what you may have been told. Yes, you do need some protein as provided in your diet programme, but a high-protein diet may overload your body with waste products. Disposing of these will divert blood away from your muscles when you exercise.

Unrefined carbohydrates are very important for fuelling your muscles with energy and giving you stamina and endurance. That's why baked potatoes, brown rice, wholemeal bread and muesli are included in the diet. These are probably the best foods that you can eat. Rich in fibre, vitamins, minerals and trace elements, they supply energy slowly, releasing a steady flow of glucose into your bloodstream. In contrast, sugar and refined carbohydrate foods flood the system with glucose and thus trigger off an insulin response. This may lead to low blood sugar levels, hunger, fatigue and irritability. Any excess glucose in the body is turned into fat. You can avoid this energy trap by choosing unrefined slow-energy release foods. That means saying 'no' to sweet drinks, white bread, cakes, biscuits, creamy desserts and chocolate.

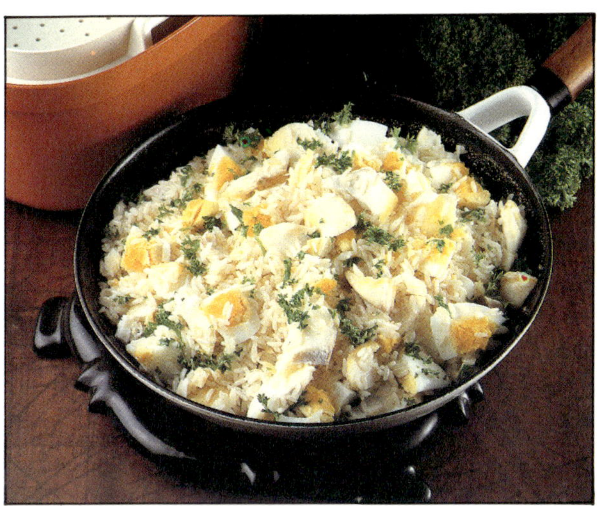

Smoked haddock kedgeree

50g/2oz long-grain rice (preferably brown)
2.5ml/½ teaspoon curry powder
100g/4oz cooked, flaked smoked haddock
1 hard-boiled egg, roughly chopped
salt and pepper
15ml/1 tablespoon chopped parsley

Cook the rice in boiling salted water until tender. Drain and mix well with the remaining ingredients. Eat with lemon wedges and a little mango chutney.

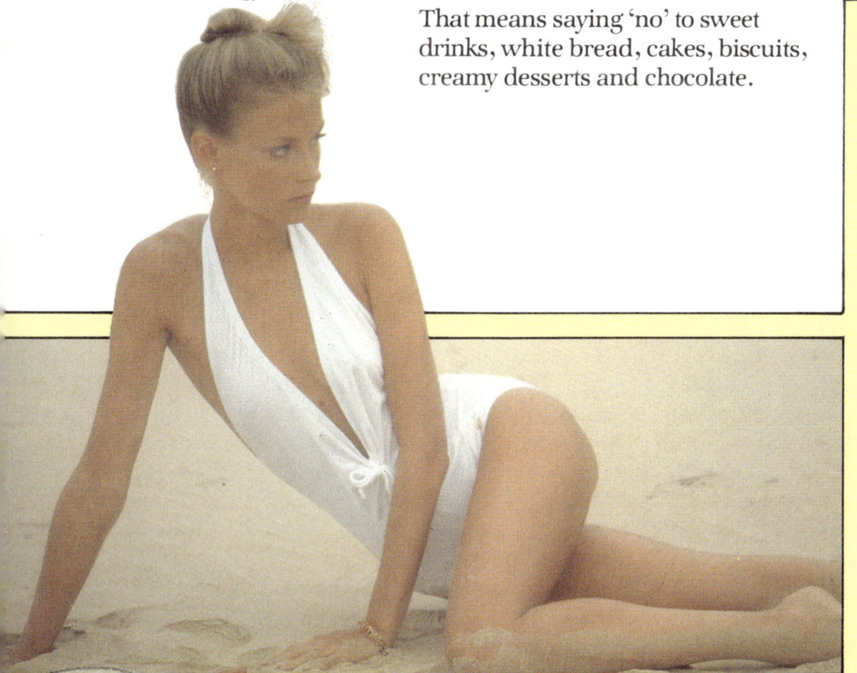

Holiday tip

If you have freckles you don't want, then you can buy a special cream to help them fade away and even out skin tone. Freckles occur when the tanning melanin granules in your skin are spaced apart and do not rise evenly to the surface. They are not the same as liver spots on hands and faces which are usually a result of too much sun coupled with the natural ageing process in your skin. Before you use a bleaching cream, however, do a patch test as it may contain irritating chemical substances. Of course, the freckles will reappear when you venture out into the holiday sunshine.

Day 10

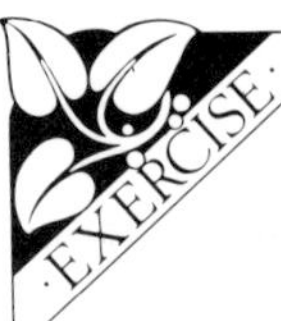

Go for a run and check up on your ideal training pulse rate

Go for a jog today but try changing your route slightly to add interest. It can get pretty boring if you always take the same roads and paths. So ring the changes by discovering new runs and different scenery. By now, you should be jogging all the time. If so, extend your time out to 20 instead of 15 minutes. You may find it more fun to run with a friend. Then you can encourage each other and chat as you run along. You may smile at this, but you should be able to hold a conversation if you are running correctly and comfortably. Don't worry if you still haven't reached this stage — just keep trying and we promise that it will get easier with practice.

You may find it useful to measure your pulse as you run along. This is a good way of checking up on how your body is responding to aerobic exercise. Most people have a resting pulse rate of 60-80 beats per minute but this increases when you run. Your heart has to beat faster to pump the oxygenated blood around your body to the muscles. You can take your pulse rate by pressing lightly on the inside of your wrist (the thumb side) with your third and fourth fingers. Count for 15 seconds and then multiply by four to determine the rate per minute. Take your pulse at rest before you run, when you are out running, and again afterwards before you wash after the cool-down stretching exercises.

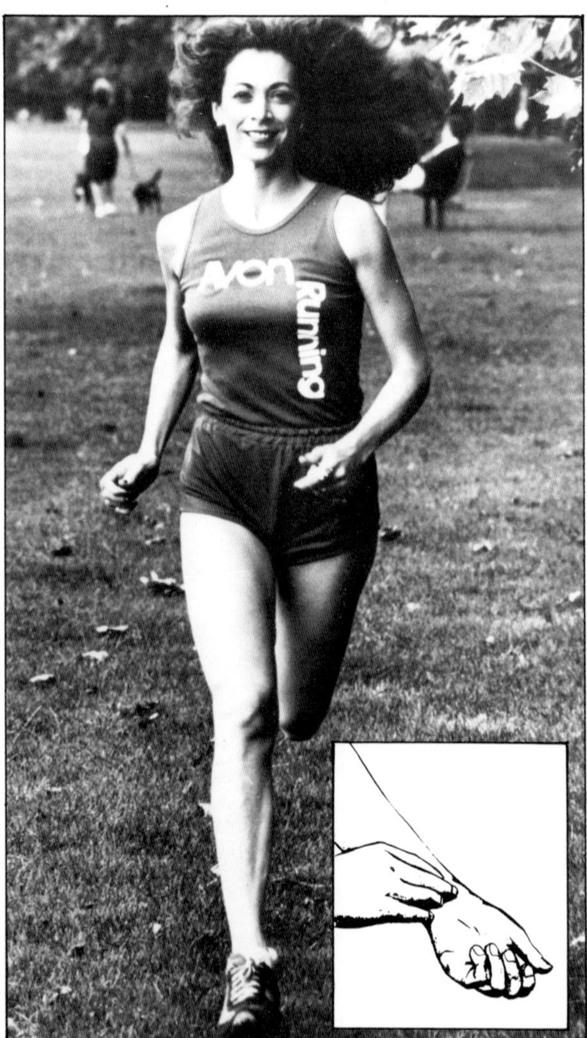

As a rough rule of thumb, your running pulse rate should fall somewhere between the maximum and minimum permissible limits. You can calculate these as follows:

1 Deduct your age from 200 to find your maximum level.

2 Deduct your age from 170 to find your minimum level. So if you are 30, your pulse rate should lie in the region of 140-170 beats per minute. Any slower and you are not pushing yourself hard enough. Any faster and you are overdoing it, so slow down. As you get more used to running and exercise in general, you will feel stronger and will find the pace that is best for you. You will also find that if running becomes a part of your life and you keep it up after the programme finishes, your pulse resting rate will slow down. This is a healthy sign that your heart is becoming stronger and more efficient.

Holiday tip

You may find it a good idea to keep a record of your progress in the exercise programme, especially at running, swimming, cycling and skipping. You can jot down your comments in a diary or notebook with details of how far you ran or cycled, how many lengths of the pool you swam or how many skips you managed and how long it took. You can even say how you felt, what your pulse rate was and whether you experienced any soreness or stiffness afterwards. You can monitor your progress in this way and set yourself new goals and challenges. Also, if you get the odd depressing day when you don't seem to be exercising at your best, you can look back through your daily log and chart your progress since Day 1 of the programme. When you see how far you have come already and how much fitter you are, you will be encouraged to continue down the road to lasting fitness and good health.

·DIET·

Discover the power of raw foods and include them in your diet

Raw foods play an important part in your diet, and it is essential that you eat a salad and some raw fruit every day. Scientists have now discovered that they play a role in fighting cancer, ulcers, high blood pressure and many other modern diseases; that they help ward off infection; and slow down the ageing process. Many top athletes now eat a diet which is high in raw foods — nuts, seeds, grains, vegetables and fruit. They find that they have more energy and give better performances.

Of course, it is not a good idea to eat a totally raw diet and become a crank, but your health and general well-being can benefit from eating some raw foods. Try starting the day with a bowl of home-made muesli embellished with chopped fresh fruit, nuts, sesame, pumpkin or sunflower seeds and a sprinkling of bran and wheatgerm. Eat a salad for lunch and fresh fruit for dinner. As you can see, it's very simple — even for someone who usually eats only cooked foods and processed convenience meals. You will discover the true flavours and textures of different foods for the first time.

There are beauty benefits, too, to be derived from raw foods. This is partly because nutrients are not destroyed or lost in the cooking process, especially the water-soluble vitamins B and C, which are essential for good skin. Freshly squeezed juices and salads every day will provide the vitamins and minerals you need for beautiful skin and hair.

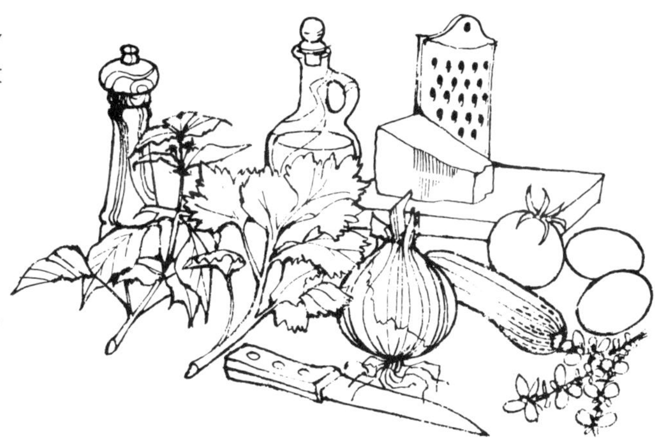

Frittata

½ onion, sliced
5ml/1 teaspoon olive oil
1 small courgette, sliced
1 large tomato, skinned and chopped
2 eggs
chopped basil, oregano, celery leaves
salt and pepper
5ml/1 teaspoon grated Parmesan cheese

Sauté onion gently in oil until soft. Add courgette and tomato and cook for a few more minutes. Beat eggs and stir in chopped herbs, seasoning and cheese. Add the cooked vegetable mixture. Cook over low heat until set and golden underneath. Place under hot grill to brown the top. Cool and eat at room temperature.

·BEAUTY·

Sports beauty — how to protect skin against the great outdoors

When you exercise, don't wear lots of thick make-up which will smudge and run when you start to perspire, nor mascara which will streak your face like a zebra crossing on a hot day. Although you want to look your best at all times, it is important to allow your skin to breathe while affording it some protection against the elements. You can buy special sports make-up products which moisturise your skin and guard against the drying effects of wind and pollution. Many of these beauty products contain a special sun filter, too. Any foundation you choose should be light and natural — you may find a tinted moisturiser more suitable.

Or you can cleanse your face thoroughly before you exercise and use your run, work-out or cycle as a beauty treatment. Physical effort raises your skin temperature and boosts circulation while opening pores so that your skin is more receptive to any deep-action cream you apply. Put some on before you exercise. Afterwards, cleanse really thoroughly to get rid of dirt, pollutants and perspiration. You will probably find that your skin becomes more active than usual when you start the exercise programme but it will soon settle down and look better than ever before.

When you're out running or cycling, you will need to protect your lips against cold winds and hot sunshine, or they may become chapped or burnt. Wear a lip balm which acts as a barrier to make sure that lips stay moist. You can wear a coloured lipstick over the top if wished. Don't choose a strong colour like deep red or orange. Go for pale silvery pink glosses which look more natural.

You probably don't need eye make-up when you're exercising, but if you are a person who feels naked without it, choose a waterproof mascara that will not run or, better still, get your eye lashes dyed.

·BEAUTY·

Taking care of your eyes means rest, good diet and exercise

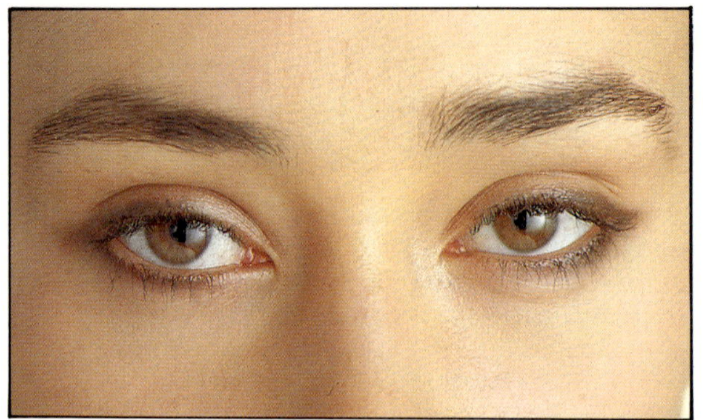

To stay healthy and strong, eyes need exercise, nutritious food and rest. Every day you should do a few simple eye exercises:

1 Roll your eyes to left and right in complete circles. Repeat 10 times.

2 Hold a pencil about 30cm/12in in front of your face and slowly move it from left to right, following it with your eyes. Now bring it to the centre and focus on it. Then look far beyond it at a distant object and after a few seconds focus on the pencil again. Repeat 5 times.

If your eyes are swollen, tired or sore, you can try out the following remedies to bring relief:

1 Lie down for 10-15 minutes with a cold tea-bag or slice of cucumber over each eye.

2 Pour a little cold witch-hazel onto two cotton wool pads and place one on each eye. Rest for 10 minutes.

If you have dark circles beneath your eyes, you might be suffering from lack of sleep, anaemia or even some minor infection. A healthy diet with plenty of vitamins A, B, C and E will help keep eyes healthy and prevent wrinkling and sagging of the skin around them. A daily salad of green and yellow fruit and vegetables and wholegrain bread will provide essential nutrients.

The skin around your eyes is very delicate, fine and prone to lines and wrinkles. From your early twenties onwards, you should apply a *little* nourishing eye cream every night before you go to bed. Moisturising and soothing, it will help plump out the skin and prevent laughter lines. If your eyes are very sensitive, try dabbing on a tiny drop of avocado, apricot or almond oil. The way in which you make-up your eyes and remove mascara is also important. Try not to wrinkle up your forehead when concentrating on colouring your lashes and go for a non-waterproof mascara which is easier to remove. Strong removers can irritate the skin on lids and may even damage very delicate tissues. Opt for a gentle non-oily remover.

·EXERCISE·

Work-out with weights for a better, firmer body shape

For a complete change, try working-out with weights today to improve muscle tone and make you generally firmer and leaner. Don't worry about developing rippling, bulging muscles and becoming 'Superwoman'. Women can't build muscle bulk like men because of their hormonal make-up. If you practise weight-training with light weights, say, 1.25kg/2½lb, you can slim down the heavy areas of your body and maintain or increase areas which need more mass. You don't need special dumb-bells. You can improvise with soup or beer cans or even telephone directories. Wear something loose and comfortable — shorts and T-shirt or a light tracksuit — to allow unrestricted movement.

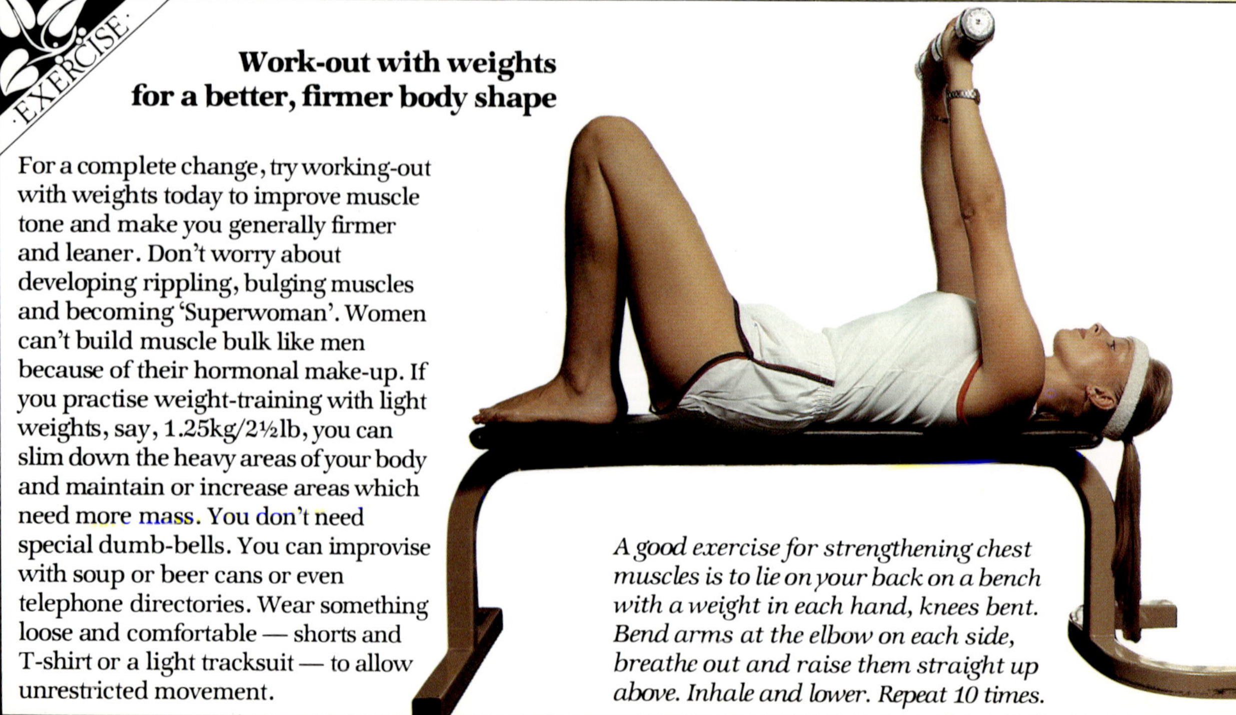

A good exercise for strengthening chest muscles is to lie on your back on a bench with a weight in each hand, knees bent. Bend arms at the elbow on each side, breathe out and raise them straight up above. Inhale and lower. Repeat 10 times.

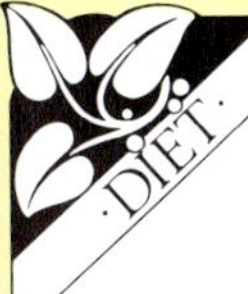

Discover the power of live sprouted beans in salads and omelettes

Sprouted beans, grains and seeds are a good source of vegetable protein and vitamins B and C. They add flavour, nutritional goodness and a crisp, crunchy texture to salads and are easy to grow yourself. You can experiment with mung beans (the familiar Chinese bean sprouts), alfalfa seeds, lentils, chick peas, buckwheat and soya beans. Just buy untreated seeds, beans or grains at your local health food store and place a heaped large spoonful in a jam jar with enough warm water to cover them. Leave overnight and the next day, cover with a piece of muslin secured with a rubber band. Drain off the water through the muslin and cover again with fresh warm water. Place the jar on a light airy windowsill which should be warm but *not* hot. Later in the day, rinse the beans or seeds yet again in more fresh water.

Continue rinsing the beans in warm water twice daily until the sprouts are sufficiently large to use in salads (takes 3-6 days). They are excellent served with an avocado dressing in salads, or use as a filling for omelettes and wholemeal pitta bread pouches.

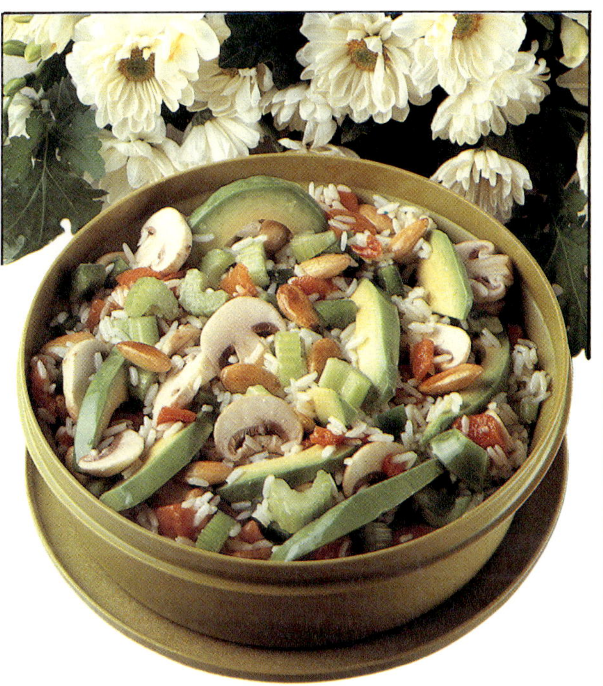

Rice and avocado salad

50g/2oz long-grain rice (preferably brown)
1 stick celery, sliced
50g/2oz button mushrooms, sliced
¼ red pepper, diced
¼ green pepper, diced
25g/1oz almonds
½ small avocado, peeled and sliced
squeeze lemon juice and little oil

Cook the rice in boiling salted water. Drain and mix well with celery, mushrooms, diced pepper and almonds. Add avocado and gently toss in lemon juice and some olive oil (as little as possible).

Side bends

1 *Stand with left arm bent behind head. Lean over, holding weight in right hand. Straighten up.*
2 *Repeat 10 times and then change sides for 10.*

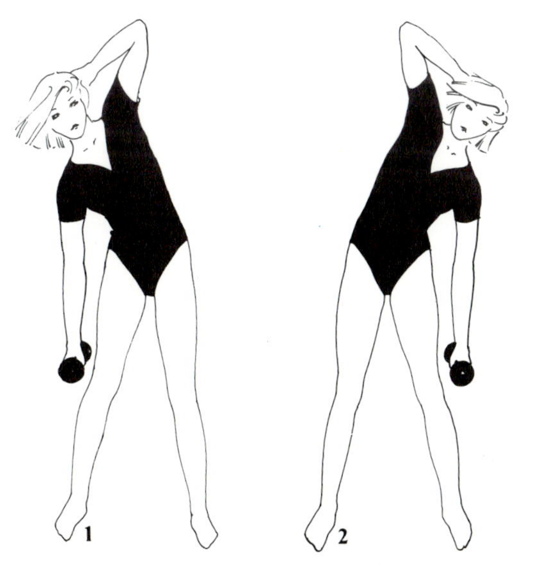

Holiday tip

Take up a new sport like tennis, squash or badminton. They all involve flexibility and bursts of speed and power. They will make your exercise programme more interesting and fun. If you don't know the rules and strokes or haven't played for several years, it is a good idea to take a beginner's or refresher course to brush up on the basics. Unlike the physical activities slotted into the exercise programme, all these sports require a partner/opponent. You can either join a club or go to your local sports centre — most have their own courts.

Day 12

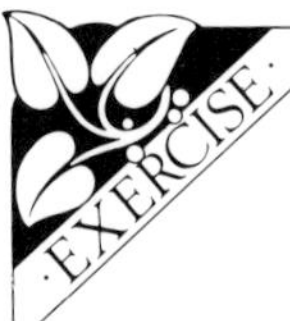

Work yourself hard for a slimmer, firmer behind

It's work-out time again so roll out a mat or blanket for the floor exercises and put on a leotard or shorts and T-shirt. Turn on the record player to a strong disco beat and go through your usual routine — warm-up, upper arms, waist, abdominals, hips and thighs — and then add some new exercises. Today, the emphasis is on buttocks and getting your bottom into shape for your holiday swimsuit. Running and cycling will go a long way towards firming up and trimming a large behind but these exercises will really work the muscles hard. Practise them every day if this is a problem area for you, and you will soon find that you can fit into a tighter pair of jeans or a minute bikini with ease.

Buttock lifts

1 *Lie on your back, feet on the ground hip distance apart and arms at your sides, palms flat.*

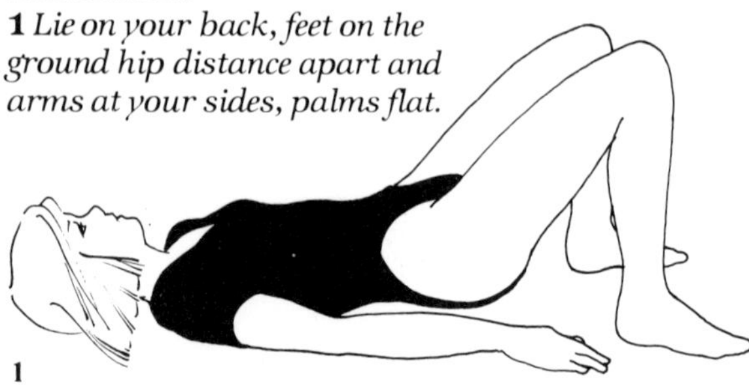

1

2 *Raise your buttocks slightly off the floor, squeeze hard, hold for a count of five and then release as you lower them. Don't touch down. Repeat the exercise 20 times.*

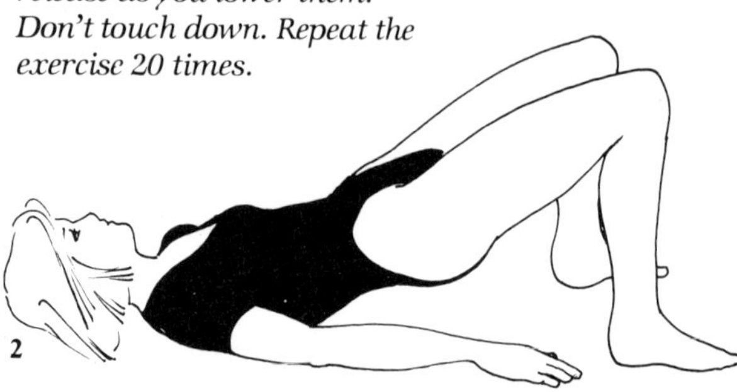

2

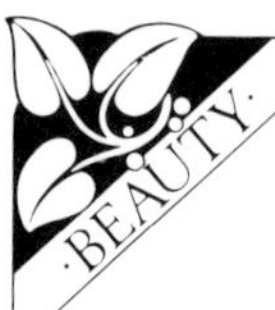

Learn how to relax with some soothing deep-breathing exercises

Try out some breathing techniques which will help you feel restful and eliminate any tension from your mind and body. You might think that breathing comes so naturally that you know how to do it without being told, but most people do not breathe correctly. Because they exhale in shallow breaths and not fully enough they retain some of the waste materials they inhale in their bodies. Over a long period of time, these can contribute towards chest disorders, premature ageing and disease. Quick shallow breathing, especially when you're angry or tired prevents sufficient oxygen entering your bloodstream, but slow, deep breathing supplies more oxygen to meet your body's needs, expels waste products and carbon-dioxide and makes you feel calmer and more relaxed.

Good breathing is also vitally important whenever you exercise. Take deep breaths right from your abdomen, inhaling through your nose and exhaling through your mouth. Keep breathing evenly and deeply to maintain a steady flow of oxygen to your muscles. This will help you to run or cycle more effortlessly and to attack your work-out programme more easily, too. Here are some deep-breathing exercises for you to try. Practised regularly, they are a good beauty aid as they will help supply your skin with more oxygen for cell metabolism.

1 Lie flat on your back on the floor, arms at your sides and palms upwards. Inhale deeply and slowly all the way down to your abdomen until your lungs are fully expanded. Hold it and count to five slowly. Then gradually exhale and relax. Repeat five times. If you are doing it properly, you should be able to feel your abdomen rise when you breathe in and fall as you breathe out.

2 Sit cross-legged on the floor with your back straight, arms held behind you. Slowly inhale through your nose, rotating your head slowly forwards and then round over your right shoulder, backwards and then forwards over your left shoulder to complete a full circle. Now slowly exhale and repeat the exercise in the opposite direction. Relax.

These exercises will help you to develop greater lung capacity. Practise them every day and you will soon feel generally more relaxed and fresher, too, as more oxygen flows to the cells and more waste and toxins are expelled from your body.

DIET

Kick the sugar habit and use more natural sweeteners

Most people seem to have a sweet tooth and find many unsweetened dishes and drinks unpalatable, yet sugar is a major cause of dental decay and diabetes and is best left out of your everyday diet and reserved for special occasions only. It is fashionable to use brown sugar instead of white, but although this contains more minerals it is still just as damaging and is virtually empty calories. Sugar-laden products are often advertised as being good for athletes because they contain glucose which provides us with energy, but it is better to get your energy from other more nutritious, less unhealthy foods such as wholemeal bread, brown rice and other unrefined carbohydrates.

You should also be aware that sugar is often disguised in products under names such as sucrose, fructose, glucose, dextrose, maltose and corn syrup. These are all synonyms for sugar — look out for them on food labels and pass them by in favour of unsweetened products. You can use honey and molasses as sweeteners, but although they are rich in mineral goodness, they are high in calories. Probably the best way to sweeten muesli, desserts and cakes is to make use of dried fruit — dates, sultanas, raisins, currants, dried apricots, prunes and figs.

If you cannot bear unsweetened tea and coffee, you may find yourself reaching automatically for some artificial, low-calorie sweetener. However, doctors and scientists are worried that some of these products may be potentially harmful so they are best avoided, too. If you cut down on sugar gradually — for instance, reducing your sugar intake in tea from two spoonfuls to one and later to a half — you will soon be able to kick the habit altogether and enjoy the real flavour of food for the first time.

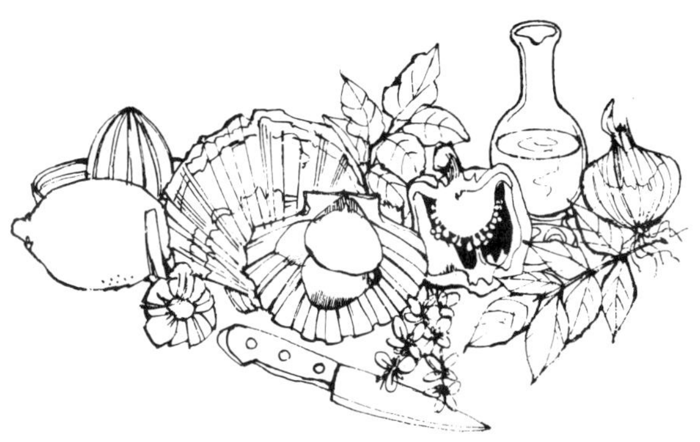

Seafood kebabs

100g/4oz scallops or white fish, cut in chunks
15ml/1 tablespoon oil
juice of ½ lemon
1 clove garlic, crushed
chopped fresh oregano or basil
½ red pepper, cut in chunks
1 small onion, quartered
1 bay leaf

If using scallops, poach gently in a little water for 3-4 minutes and drain. Place fish or scallops in dish and pour over oil, lemon, garlic and herbs. Cover and leave in refrigerator for several hours. Thread scallops or fish onto kebab skewers with pepper, onion and bay leaf. Brush with remaining marinade and grill, turning if necessary, until cooked (about 10 minutes).

Holiday tip

You need a good night's sleep to relax your body and mind, rejuvenate tired skin and recharge your energy. The amount of sleep you need is entirely individual and may vary from five to nine hours a day. Your body will adjust itself automatically to what is best for it. If you have difficulty sleeping, try one of the following: step up your level of exercise; don't drink coffee or alcohol before going to bed; have a warm, relaxing bath last thing; have a soothing cup of herb tea; sleep in a cool room with a window open; use ear plugs to keep out noise; and, most important, establish a regular bedtime routine and time.

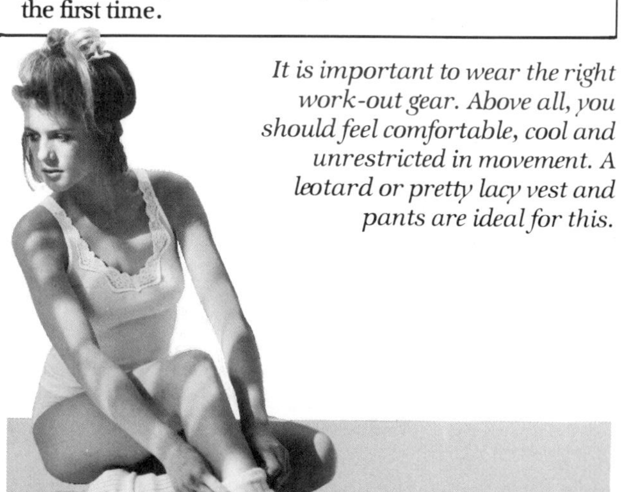

It is important to wear the right work-out gear. Above all, you should feel comfortable, cool and unrestricted in movement. A leotard or pretty lacy vest and pants are ideal for this.

Day 13

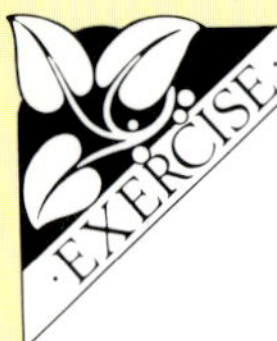

Stretch out and relax with yoga

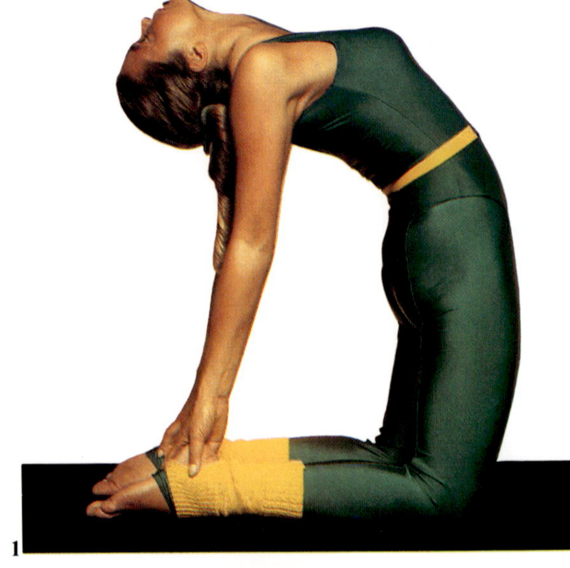

Your exercise programme hits a different note today. Instead of your usual strenuous routine, try stretching out your muscles very slowly with some yoga. This is a unique combination of relaxation and exercise and although it may seem very slow and easy after running or working-out, it is exercising your muscles but in a different way. Followers of yoga claim that it can increase suppleness, diminish tension and bring peace of mind, making you better able to cope with the daily pressures of modern living. The key to successful yoga is to perform the exercises *(asanas)* gently and slowly without straining. Never bounce into a given position or use fast, jerky movements. Gently stretch until you reach the desired position. Then hold it as long as you can — until you feel any discomfort — and slowly come out of the stretch back to the starting position. Here are some asanas for you to try:

1

1 The camel
Kneeling with knees shoulder width apart and arms at sides, inhale and bend backwards over legs. Grasp heels and move stomach forwards. Hold for 5.

2

2 The plough
Lie down with arms at sides. Extend legs over head until touching floor. Hold as long as you can.

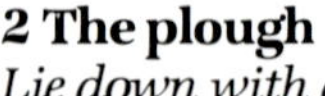

The bow
Lie face down and bend right leg, clasping foot with right hand. Do the same with left foot. Slowly raise chest and thighs off floor. Stretch out head and neck and rock gently to and fro, breathing very deeply.

BEAUTY

Let your skin breathe with a deep-cleansing facial sauna

Give your face a deep cleansing treatment today with a herbal steam infusion. All you need is a basin, some boiling hot water, a towel and a small bundle of fresh herbs. This facial sauna helps open the pores in your skin and draws out any dirt, pollutants and impurities so that your skin feels really clean and baby soft afterwards. It is particularly effective on oily skins with enlarged blocked pores, especially if you live or work in a big city where the air is dirty and polluted with car exhaust fumes. Note that if you have broken veins and capillaries on your cheeks and nose and your skin is particularly sensitive, you would benefit more from a specially formulated face mask.

Choose from the following herbs — try to use fresh ones if possible for the best effects:

1 Dry skin: sage, comfrey or fennel

2 Oily skin: mint, camomile, nettle, basil, elder blossom or rosemary

3 Normal skin: lavender, rose petal, acacia flower or peppermint

Place the fresh herbs in a basin of freshly boiled water. Lean over the basin, with your head covered in a towel, and gently steam your face for 10 mintues. Splash with cold water and pat dry. While your skin is pink, glowing and highly receptive, gently rub in a moisturising or treatment cream.

This is an excellent way of softening skin and improving circulation, but it shouldn't be carried out more than once a week by people with dry and normal skins. If your skin is oily, you might benefit from a twice-weekly facial sauna.

Holiday tip

Treat yourself to a good pair of sunglasses which will protect your eyes from glare in bright sunshine. The quality of the lenses is more important than fashionable frames although the two tend to go together nowadays. They should be sufficiently dark to eliminate at least 70 per cent of the ultraviolet spectrum and have a scratch-resistant surface. Go for dark colours — brown, grey or green — and not pinks, blues and yellows which let too much light through. To test for quality, hold the sunglasses at arm's length and focus on a vertical object through one lens. When you move the glasses up and down the image should remain still.

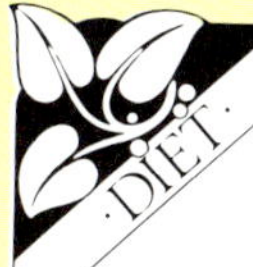

DIET

Read food labels carefully for chemical additives

Not all canned and packaged foods are bad for you as you will see if you survey the shelves of a health food store. Even some supermarket convenience foods are really quite healthy. The trick is to know how to read the labels where the ingredients are listed and to identify any culprits and potentially unhealthy additives. Some food additives can be a threat to health — for instance, they may be linked with a tendency to produce cancerous cells in the body, or they may tend to harm a foetus in a woman's womb or produce genetic changes. And although governments strive to rigorously test and regulate them, scientists and doctors still have doubts about their safety and long-term effects on our health.

Over 3000 additives are currently permitted in Great Britain alone. They are present only in minute quantities but over a period of time they can build up in the body and may be potentially toxic. The ones to look out for particularly are:

1 Sodium nitrite, found in many processed meats, sausages, cheeses.

2 BHT, a petroleum additive.

3 Red food colouring (not cochineal or vegetable colourings) but a special red dye.

These are all potential carcinogens (cancer-forming) and should be avoided wherever possible. Preservatives, emulsifiers, flavourings, colourings, stabilisers and sweeteners are all supposed to improve the appearance and flavour of food and extend its shelf life, but they may be harmful in the long run, and it is certainly a lot healthier and more enjoyable to eat natural whole food alternatives as advocated in the Diet Programme. If you are pregnant, then you should avoid additives at all costs.

Tomato and lentil salad

50g/2oz brown Continental lentils
½ small onion, chopped
1 spring onion, chopped
1 tomato, quartered
15ml/1 tablespoon olive oil
5ml/1 teaspoon wine vinegar
salt and pepper
chopped parsley and mint

Soak lentils for 1 hour. Remove any gritty pieces. Drain and cook in fresh water until tender (about 1¼ hours). Strain and mix with other ingredients.

Brush and floss for healthy teeth and gums

Daily care is vital for healthy teeth and gums. If you eat too much sugar you are a likely candidate for gum disease and tooth decay, so if you want to avoid false teeth in later life, cut out sugar *now* and make brushing and flosssing a part of your daily beauty regimen. They will help control the build-up of harmful bacteria (plaque) in your mouth and reduce the risk of decay. Brushing at least twice daily, morning and evening, will help fight plaque, but a disclosing tablet, available from most drugstores, will reveal the areas of plaque and food residue that are left even after a good brush.

Go out today and buy some dental floss — the unwaxed sort is best. After cleaning your teeth, break off a length of floss and wind each end around the first two fingers of each hand. Slide it up and down between your teeth, two at a time, to remove any food particles and plaque. Be gentle and don't hurt your gums although it is more effective if you move the floss right up into the gum crevice. Do not worry if your gums bleed initially — this will stop as they get tougher and stronger from regular flossing. Brushing, flossing and regular visits to your dentist are the only way to achieve beautiful white teeth and a dazzling smile.

Floss your teeth every day if possible. Hold floss around a finger on each hand and pull to and fro and up and down between the teeth to remove any plaque and bacteria effectively.

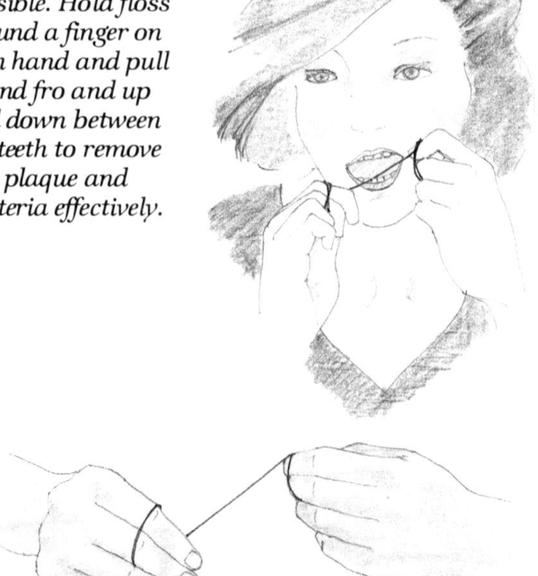

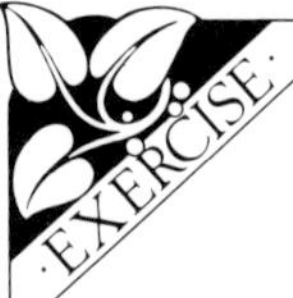

Try out some slimming pool exercises in the water

Go for a cycle or a swim today. Aim for about 30-45 minutes' cycling or 20 minutes' swimming. If you are in the swimming pool, practise some of these water exercises. They are an effective way to firm up your body and will stand you in good stead for the hotel pool when you go on holiday. If you want to look slim and shapely in your swimsuit, then you can use the water pressure to help you exercise.

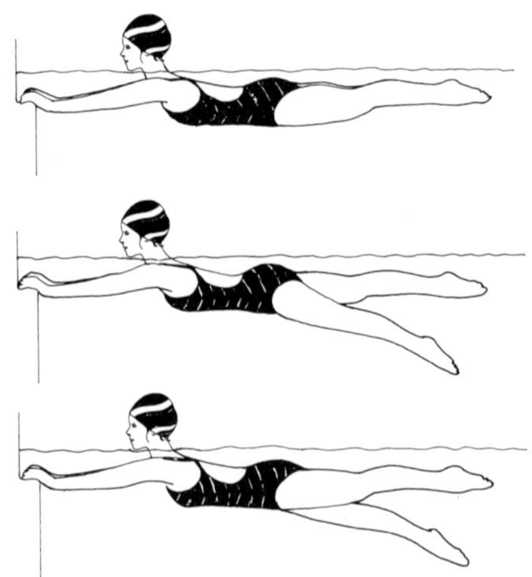

Leg kicks: *holding onto edge, float horizontally with straight legs. Keeping arms straight, kick really hard for at least 3 minutes. Rest and repeat.*

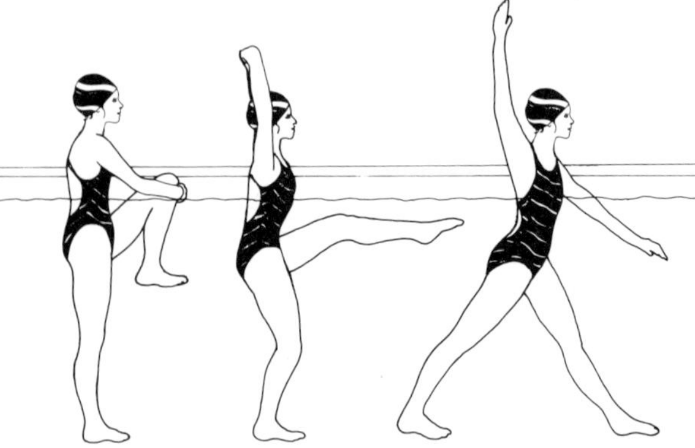

Pool walking: *stand in the shallow end of pool with one knee held up in clasped hands. Now throw arms up over head and take a big step, swing one arm down to water. Repeat with other leg. Continue for 3 minutes.*

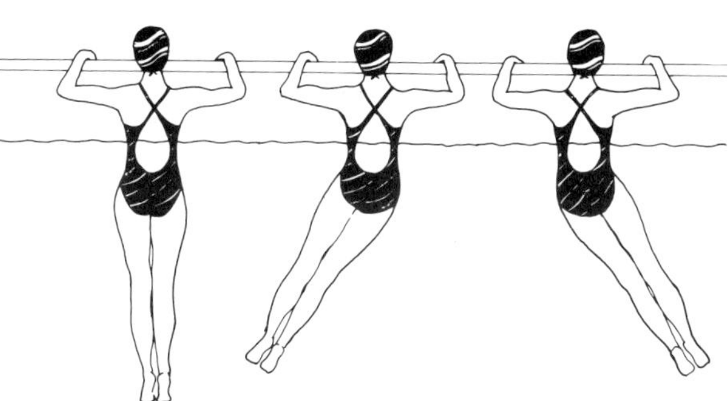

Waist toner: *holding onto edge or rail with straight legs and pointed toes, swing legs to side from waist only. Swing to other side and repeat 30 times.*

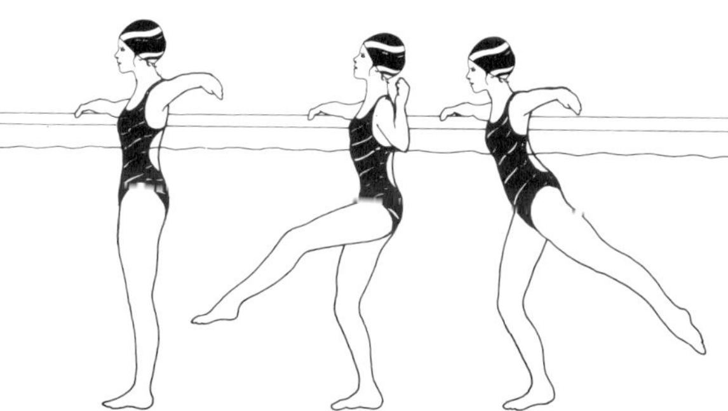

Leg strengthener: *standing on bottom of pool in the shallow end and holding onto edge or rail with one arm and the other outstretched to the side above water level, raise one leg forwards as high as it will go and then backwards equally high. It is quite hard as you are pushing against the pressure of the water. Repeat 15 times and then change legs.*

Holiday tip

If you are going abroad on a motoring holiday, check that you have a full driving licence which is valid in all the countries you intend to visit. Some require a special permit or official translation of your licence — find out from your motoring organisation. You will also need adequate insurance cover. Ask your insurance company whether you are covered to drive abroad and whether you need an international certificate of insurance (green card). Insurance policies are automatically valid throughout the EEC for citizens of member states. If you are travelling further afield you may also need a *carnet* — again, check with your motoring association.

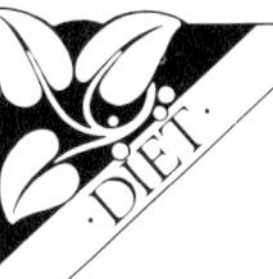

Control the amount of cholesterol in your diet

Nowadays we hear a lot about cholesterol — a sort of fat in the bloodstream which, when levels are very high, has been identified as a major factor in causing heart disease. These dangerously high cholesterol deposits are brought about by eating too many saturated fats — animal fat on meat, butter, hard margarine, cream, milk, full-fat hard cheeses and hidden fat in many processed foods — and cholesterol in foods such as eggs, meat and shellfish. This has brought about a trend towards eating a low-cholesterol diet which emphasises fish and poultry, high-fibre vegetables and fruit, and whole grains. Vegetable oils and soft polyunsaturated margarines are used in preference to hard fats and butter. Eating a healthy diet along these lines will prevent cholesterol blood levels rising too high.

However, you do need some cholesterol and your body actually synthesises it in the liver. Some substances, such as linoleic acid found in nuts and lecithin in eggs, help control and balance cholesterol levels and prevent it building up in fatty deposits on the artery walls. Sedentary people tend to have higher cholesterol levels than fit, active people irrespective of their diet, so stepping up your level of exercise will help protect your heart. If you care about your long-term health, stick to the healthy whole foods in the Diet Programme long after your holiday.

Salade nicoise

50g/2 oz stringless French beans
1 small potato
1 spring onion, chopped
1 tomato, quartered
50g/2oz canned tuna fish, drained
1 hard-boiled egg, shelled and quartered
2 black olives
15ml/1 tablespoon chopped parsley
2 anchovy fillets (optional)
salt and pepper
30ml/2 tablespoons lemony French dressing

Top and tail French beans and cook until tender. Keep pan uncovered to preserve lovely green colour. Drain andcool. Peel potato and cook until tender. Cool and cut into chunks. Mix beans and potato with the other ingredients and toss well in the dressing so everything is well-coated.

Holiday haircare

Holiday hair should be easy-to-manage and in good condition if it is to withstand the bombardment from sun, sea and wind — all of which can wreak havoc with your hair, making it dry, dull and brittle. Get your hair in good shape before you go away by visiting the hairdresser and using a deep-action conditioner. Here's how.

Choosing a summer style
A shorter cut often makes hair more manageable and easier to care for in the sun. It is cooler in hot weather, will dry naturally without a hairdryer, curling tongs or heated rollers and looks sporty, too — just right for a fortnight on the beach. Longer hair can be pinned up by day with colourful combs and slides to keep it off your shoulders and face. Leaf through some magazines to find a style you like or ask your hairdresser what she recommends. Above all, don't opt for anything fussy which is difficult and time-consuming to keep neat and tidy. Styling and drying are inevitably more difficult on holiday. Take a good look at your hair and decide whether you are happy or bored with it, whether it is in good condition and how much time you can spare to look after it well.

Feeding your hair
Your hair needs feeding from inside and outside to keep it in tip-top condition. A course of pre-holiday conditioning treatments, either at a salon or at home, are a good investment. Conditioners help protect your hair by sealing the hair shaft, filling in any splits and giving it a smooth surface. They can be used to treat dry, brittle hair and to make combing gentler and easier. If your hair is in good condition, it should be easy to care for, feel silky and look glossy and thicker.

You can feed your hair from within and improve its overall condition by sticking to the diet programme. Fresh wholefood ingredients like whole grains, fruit and vegetables all contain nutritional goodness which helps improve the quality of hair. For your hair reflects your inner state of health — if it is dull and lifeless, then you are probably unfit and under the weather. The B-complex vitamins are especially beneficial, so take brewers yeast tablets daily.

Special effects
On holiday when hair can become a problem, a soft perm may help to hold a short cut or add bounce to long, unruly hair. Drying and setting are easy as you can often just towel-dry hair, running your fingers through it for a natural look. But you must use a specially formulated perm shampoo and conditioner to keep in moisture and prevent dryness. Sun hair also looks good when streaked or highlighted. It will probably go lighter in the sun anyway so why not brighten up your image and show off your tan with some subtle highlights? For the best results, go to a professional rather than try to do it yourself at home. Remember, though, that if your hair has been chemically treated, it will need extra protection from the sun.

Hair in the sun
Just like your skin, your hair contains protective pigments which help shield it from the sun. Whereas olive skins tan more easily than fair complexions, brunettes have more built-in hair protection than blondes. In the same way that hair can be damaged and split by using an over-hot electric hairdryer, it can be scorched by the sun. To prevent it from becoming dull, dry and brittle, you need to protect it with deep-action conditioners and special hair-shield products which are now on sale in most drugstores.

To keep hair healthy, follow these basic rules when you return to your hotel room after a day on the beach:
1 Wash your hair with a mild shampoo to remove any traces of sand, sea-water or chlorinated pool water. Choose a shampoo which is based on natural ingredients, such as jojoba, apricot oil or herbs.
2 After rinsing, massage a good conditioner into the hair and scalp and leave for the specified time.
3 If necessary, use a setting gel or mousse to control flyaway hair and avoid styling problems.
4 Dry naturally if possible, or use a compact dual-voltage travel hairdryer if you are in a hurry.
5 For summer evenings, use a light hair spray to hold the style if necessary.
You can lighten blonde hair or brighten dark hair by

1

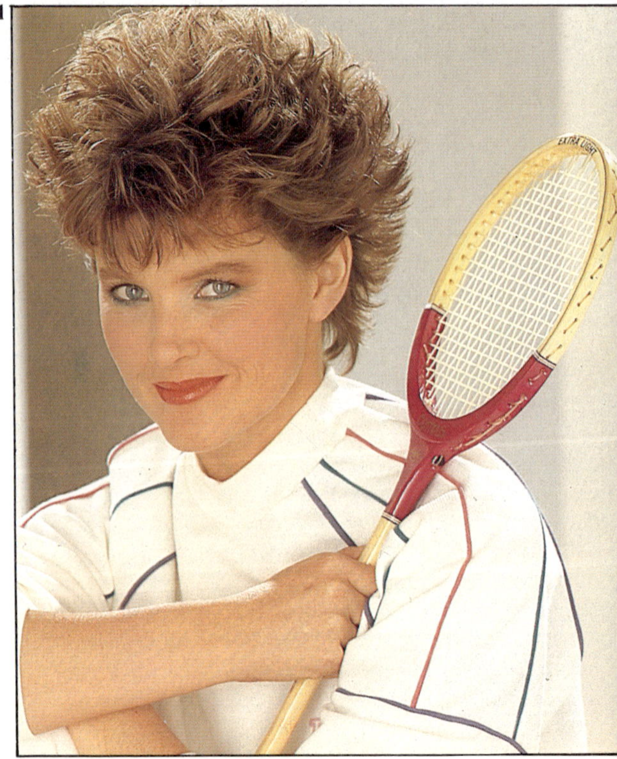

adding fresh lemon juice to the rinsing water. Rinse again and allow to dry naturally in the sun. In the morning before you venture out onto the beach you can use a special sunshield to protect your hair during the coming day. Alternatively, wear a sunhat or wrap your hair up in a colourful scarf. When swimming, use a bathing cap, or rinse hair out afterwards with fresh water. You can take some with you in a plastic bottle, or use a freshwater beach shower. Then towel-dry hair gently — never rub vigorously or you may damage the ends and cuticles.

Hair burns more easily when wet because of the reflection of ultra-violet rays off the water. Wear a fashionable swim cap — it will protect your hair and prevent possible ear infections. If you dislike wearing a cap, however, then use a special hair protection product or even wipe any excess sun tan lotion on your hands gently over your hair for added protection. Follow these basic rules and your hair can still be your crowning glory, even on holiday.

Choose a hair style to suit your lifestyle. If you play a lot of sports, a short hair cut (1) is probably the best. Away on holiday, a fashionably short crop is cool in the sun and ideal for swimming (2), while long hair can be plaited to keep it off the face (3). Permed hair, rubbed dry with a towel, still looks good (4).

2

3

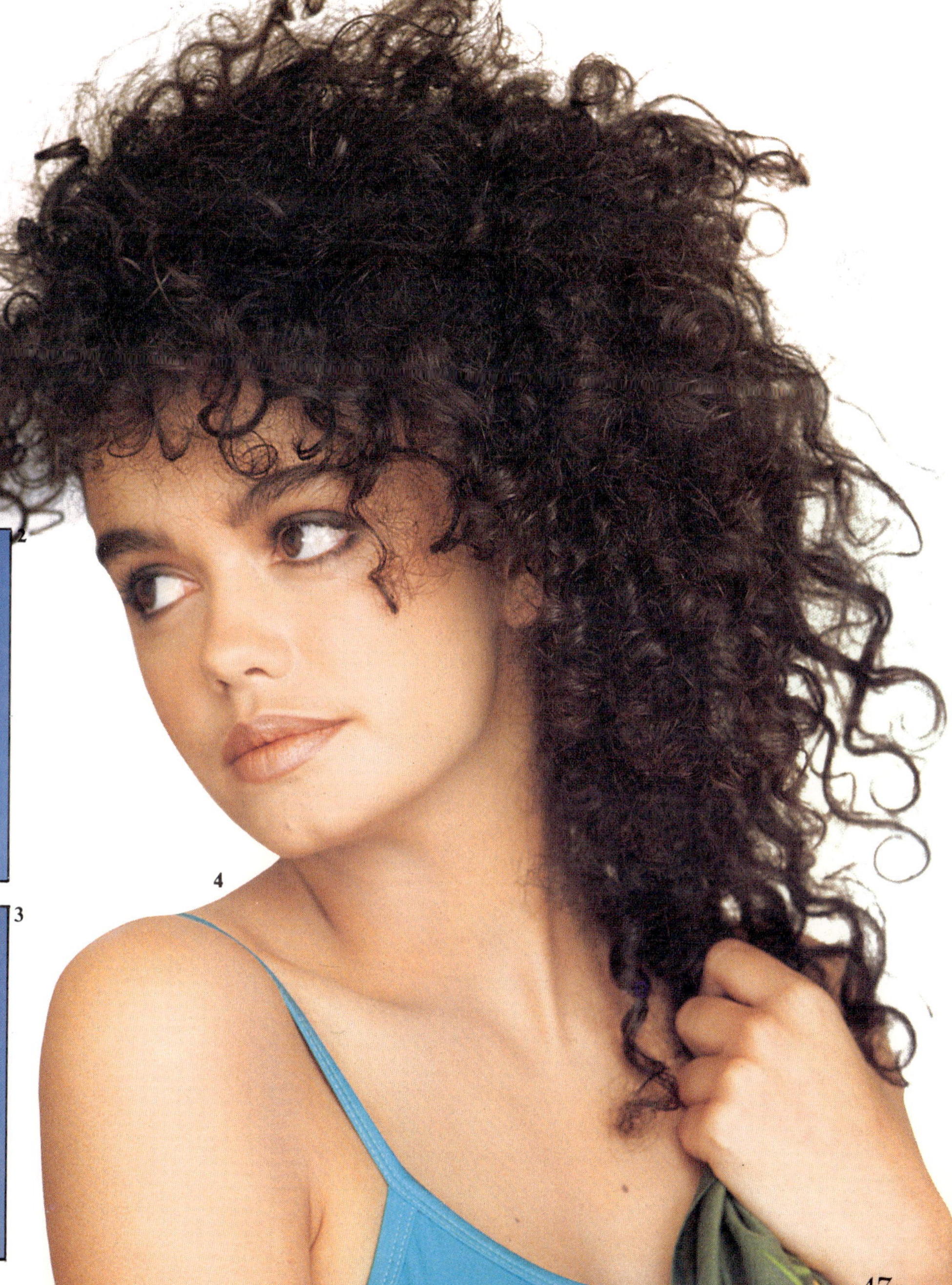

4

Day 15

·EXERCISE·

Add some new leg exercises to your work-out

Extend your work-out today with some more advanced exercises. Go through your usual work-out routine, and add these new exercises at the end before you cool-down and rest. Make sure when you work-out that you work evenly on both sides of your body. Many people work harder on one side than the other although they are quite unconscious of the fact that they are doing so, and this produces uneven results.

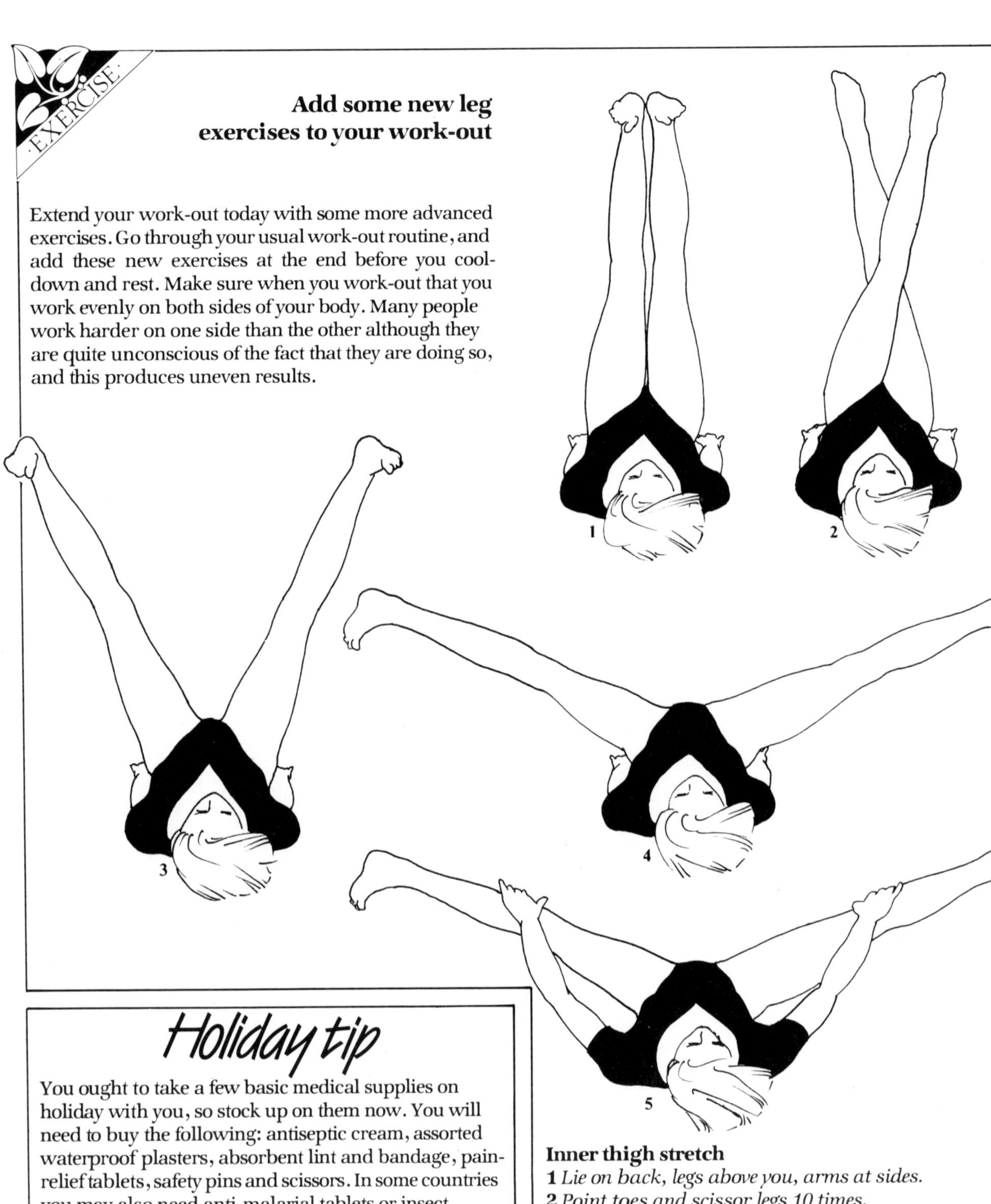

Holiday tip

You ought to take a few basic medical supplies on holiday with you, so stock up on them now. You will need to buy the following: antiseptic cream, assorted waterproof plasters, absorbent lint and bandage, pain-relief tablets, safety pins and scissors. In some countries you may also need anti-malarial tablets or insect repellant. Water-purification tablets are a safe standby for some parts of the Mediterranean, North Africa and Asia. If you tend to get holiday tummy upsets, make sure you pack some anti-diarrhoeal mixture, too.

Inner thigh stretch

1 *Lie on back, legs above you, arms at sides.*
2 *Point toes and scissor legs 10 times.*
3 *Open legs very slowly as far as possible.*
4 *Slowly bounce them up and down twice.*
5 *Push down with hands and bounce twice.*
Repeat the exercise 3 times.

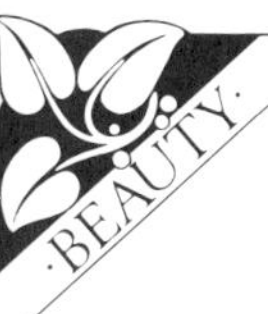

The eyes have it — aim for a natural look

Focus on your eyes today. Start by looking at your eyebrows — are they too thick, too long or too shaggy? You can improve the shape by plucking but do not overdo it — the finished look should be natural and just right for your face.

1 Gently rub a little moisturiser into the skin around your eyebrows.

2 Brush the brows into shape and start plucking any stray hairs below the main brows or in the centre above the bridge of your nose. Never pluck above the eyebrow — always from below.

3 When you have removed any straggling hairs and have achieved your desired shape, dab a little astringent toner over the area.

You can accentuate and shape your eyebrows further with eye pencils but never use heavy dark lines. Choose a colour one shade lighter than your normal hair colouring and use soft feathery strokes. Then brush your eyebrows for a more natural effect. Aim to define the eyebrow without changing its basic form.

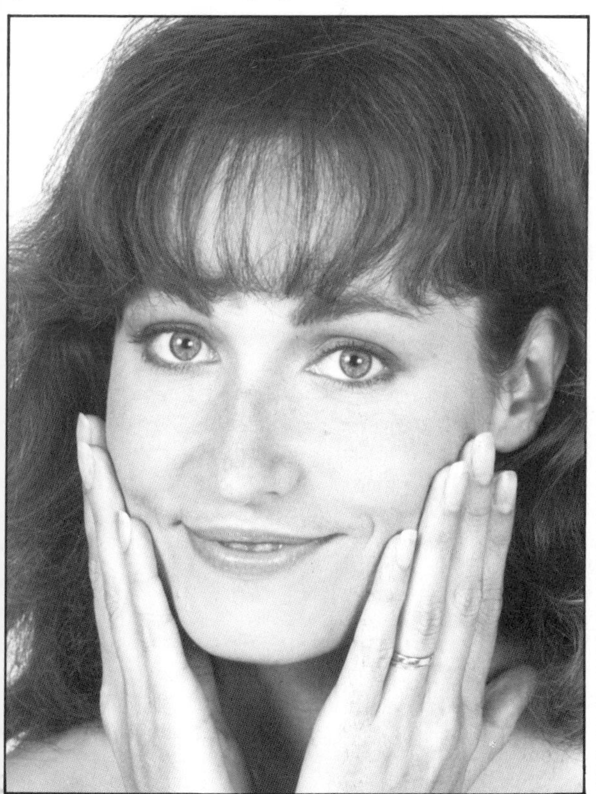

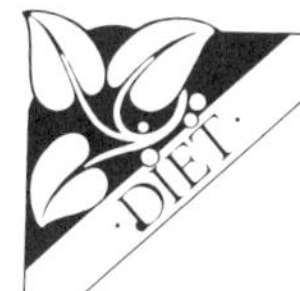

Create some colourful, healthy summer salads

Have fun experimenting with unusual salads and forget about those limp lettuce leaves, drying cucumber and soggy tomato. Instead, try mixing traditional salad vegetables with nuts, fresh fruit, beans and seeds. There are lots of vegetables which you may not have thought of eating raw: sliced button mushrooms, shredded white and red cabbage, garden peas, tiny young broad beans, grated carrot, spinach leaves and fennel. Many fresh fruits blend well with salads, especially sliced oranges, grapefruit, peaches and nectarines, apple, pears, grapes and even raspberries, strawberries and redcurrants. Add sunflower, pumpkin or sesame seeds, shelled nuts and chopped fresh herbs. You will have one of the healthiest summer salads possible.

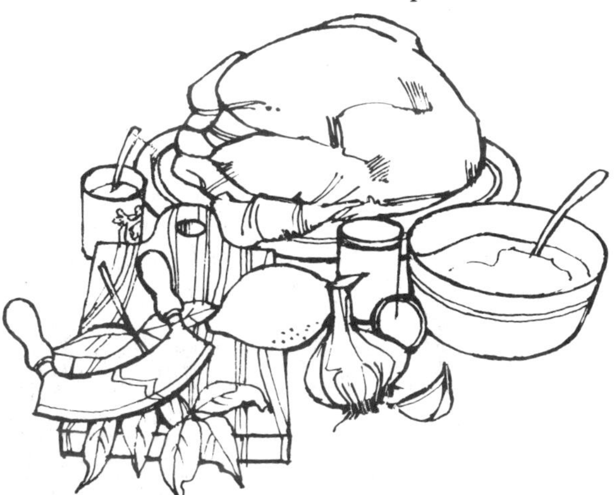

Tandoori chicken dip

juice ½ lemon
1 clove garlic, crushed
75ml/3floz natural yoghurt
good pinch ground cumin and coriander
¼ teaspoon each paprika and ginger
pinch English mustard powder
1 large or 2 small chicken breasts
Dip:
50ml/2floz natural yoghurt
few chives and fresh mint, chopped

Mix together lemon, garlic, yoghurt, spices and mustard. Cut chicken into chunks and marinate in yoghurt mixture in sealed container in refrigerator for 2-3 hours. Thread onto skewers and grill until cooked, turning. Serve with yoghurt dip mixed with herbs.

Day 16

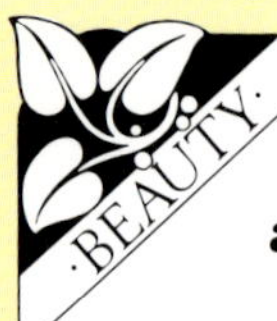

Check your posture and attack a double chin with facial massage

Bad posture is a major cause of back ache and may also lead to foot problems, fatigue, poor breathing and bad digestion. Stooping and slouching do not bode well for good looks, either, and you will look taller and slimmer when you stand and walk straight with your stomach and buttocks tucked in, and your shoulders relaxed — they don't have to be straight and held high like a guardsman's on parade.

Test your natural posture and your spine by looking at yourself sideways in a full length mirror. You should not have an exaggerated curve in your spine nor should your stomach be thrust too far forwards or your shoulders held unnaturally stiff. Get into the good posture habit — the more aware you are of the way you stand and sit, the more naturally it will come so that eventually you will not even have to think about it. If you don't carry your body and spine correctly, the vertebrae may eventually become compressed, causing friction and tension and even joint or bone displacement. Don't let this happen to you. Good posture will strengthen your back muscles and help avoid any problems.

Your profile will look even better minus a double chin. You can attack this with regular exercises, especially neck stroking and the ceiling kiss shown here. This will help break down fat and tone up and tighten neck muscles. To massage your neck, use a little vegetable or flower oil and lightly move your fingers over the skin, stroking the neck first, working upwards and outwards with both hands from front to back under the chin. Stroke firmly under the chin outwards to the jaw line. Then tap your fingertips lightly across your chin and jaw. Repeat several times each day. You can use a nourishing or moisturising cream, if wished, so that the skin can absorb its active ingredients.

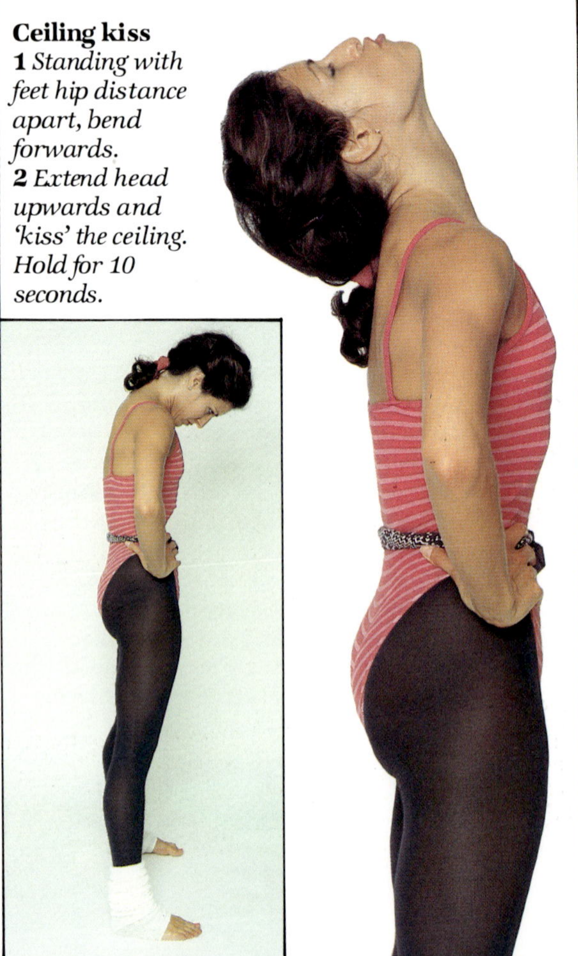

Ceiling kiss
1 *Standing with feet hip distance apart, bend forwards.*
2 *Extend head upwards and 'kiss' the ceiling. Hold for 10 seconds.*

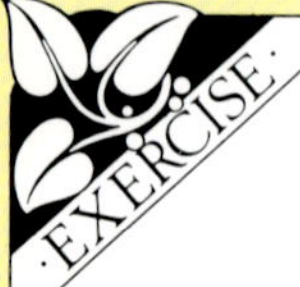

Go for a run and do some stool-stepping

More jogging today, so put on your tracksuit and running shoes and off you go for a 20 minute run/walk session after doing your usual warm-up stretches. By now you should be running a little easier and more confidently with fewer aches and pains. If you keep it up, you should be able to run two or three miles without stopping after a couple of months of training three or four times a week. But do not try to rush your progress and do it all at once — it cannot be said enough times that you should be patient and build up gradually or you may get injured and put all your earlier training in jeopardy. Respect your body and listen to what it tells you. Respond to its early warning signals when you are overdoing it before you strain a muscle or get over-tired.

Stool-stepping: this exercise will build up muscular strength and stamina. Use a stool or chest, the bottom step of the staircase or even a strong box. Step up and down again as many times as you possibly can, maintaining a steady pace. When you get breathless, pause for a rest and then repeat the exercise once more when you feel more comfortable and have recovered your breath. Try doing this every day.

DIET

Fill the shelves of your store-cupboard with healthy foods

Your larder does not have to be stocked with unhealthy packet foods, sugary jams and jellies and preservative-laden cans. You can buy healthy alternatives in health food stores. Always keep plenty of brown rice and wholemeal pasta in store; buckwheat, oats, rye flakes, millet and dried beans; dried fruits and canned fruit in natural juice, not sugary syrup. Buy canned tuna and salmon in brine, not oil; and try out some of the delicious instant vegetarian rissole mixes if you are in a great hurry. Use carob powder instead of cocoa or cooking chocolate; and look for coffee substitutes and skimmed milk powder. Other handy, healthy items to have in store include: different flavoured honeys, unsalted nuts, seeds (pumpkin, sesame, sunflower), a good range of spices and dried herbs , whole grain semolina and pudding rice, plenty of wholemeal flour and molasses.

Then you can always whisk up a snack or meal using store-cupboard ingredients as well as fresh fruit and vegetables, supplemented with poultry or fish from the freezer. You can even buy sugarless or low-sugar diabetic jams. Other useful foods are canned olives, sardines, anchovies, mussels, lumpfish roe (looks and even tastes like caviare to the uninitiated), canned bean sprouts and water chestnuts for Chinese wok cookery, and plenty of fresh free-range eggs. These are perfect for whipping up soufflés and omelettes, crêpes and vegetable quiches in a wholemeal crust.

Holiday tip

Now is the time to visit the dentist for a check-up if you haven't already done so in the last six months. Teeth should be checked regularly for cavities and signs of decay to stop the rot in time. You may be surprised to learn that most dentists are not the frightening sadists you imagine them to be. A pain-killing injection will deaden the pain of the drill and make the whole process bearable. If you want to avoid the misery of holiday toothache, it is best to have your teeth checked now. If any fillings or other work are necessary, they can be done before you leave. Ask your dentist also to clean your teeth. This involves removing plaque — the invisible bacteria and food residues which can build up despite careful brushing and ultimately lead to gum disease and tooth loss. You will be amazed at how clean and white your teeth will look.

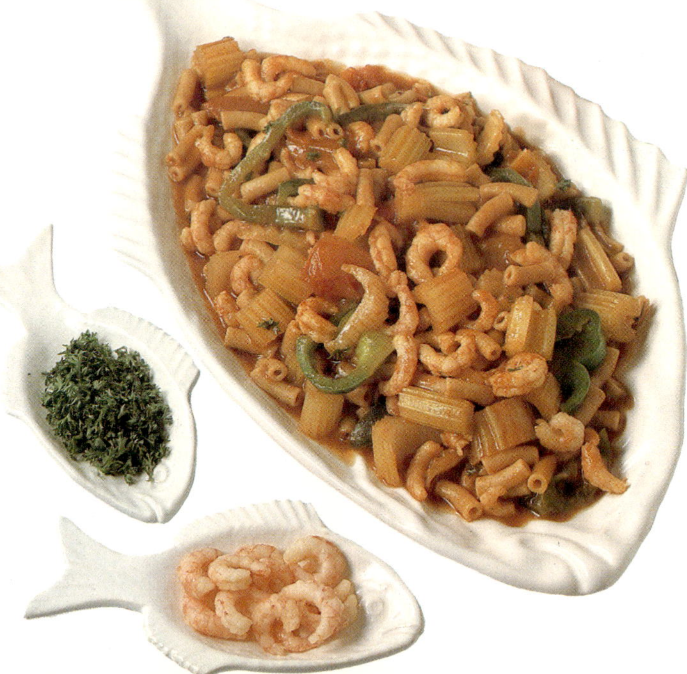

Pasta and prawn creole

½ small onion, chopped
1 stick celery, chopped
½ green pepper, cut in strips
1 clove garlic, crushed
15ml/1 tablespoon oil
175g/6oz canned tomatoes
75ml/3floz white wine or stock
15ml/1 tablespoon tomato purée
salt and pepper
50g/2oz wholewheat macaroni
75g/3oz peeled prawns

Fry onion, celery, pepper and garlic in oil until tender. Add canned tomatoes, wine, tomato purée and seasoning. Simmer 5 minutes. Add macaroni and prawns. Cover and simmer until pasta is tender and *al dente* (to 'the bite'). This takes about 15 minutes. Sprinkle with chopped parsley.

Day 17

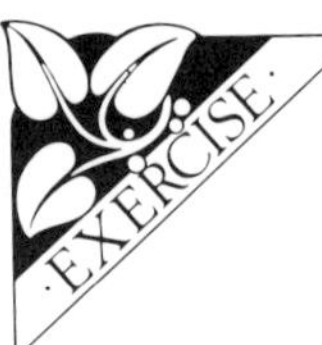

Include some aerobics in your home work-out

You do not have to go out running, swimming or cycling to benefit from aerobics. You can do it at home with these simple exercises. They will raise your pulse rate and help the blood carry more oxygen to your muscles. If you include them in your work-out routine, do them immediately after the warm-up before you go on to individual exercises. Remember to breathe deeply and evenly all the time and slow down and rest immediately you feel breathless or giddy. Start off with some room-running to warm up and get your heart beating faster.

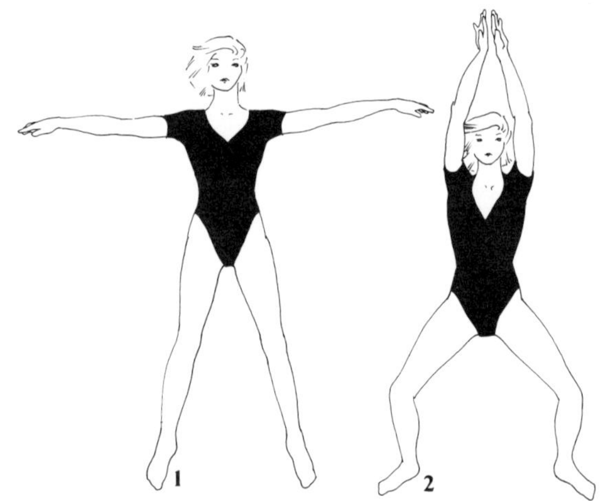

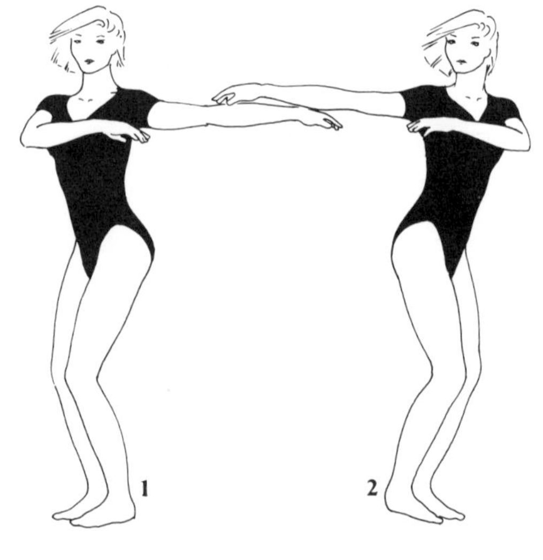

Jumping jacks (above)
1 *Standing with feet shoulder distance apart, jump with arms outstretched at shoulder height to sides.*
2 *Land with knees bent, arms raised. Repeat 20 times.*

Twisting jumps (left)
1 *Jump to one side, twisting your body to the left and throwing out your arms to the right.*
2 *Now reverse, jumping to the right and throwing out your arms to the left. Repeat 20 times.*

Heels and knees up (below)
1 *and* **2** *Run on spot lifting up heels for 10 counts.*
3 *and* **4** *Run on spot lifting up knees for 10 counts. Clap your hands as you do so. Repeat sequence.*

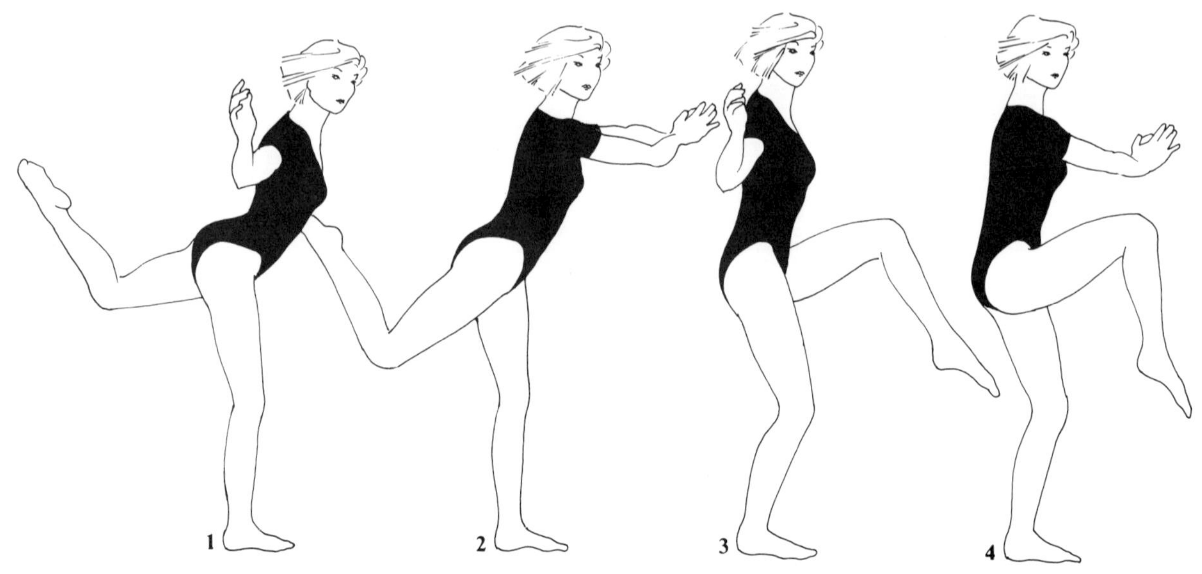

Practise a complete make-up routine in 10 mintues

Develop your own fast summer make-up routine. You don't want to spend a long time getting ready on sunny holiday mornings so you need to streamline your beauty regimen. When you get up, cleanse, tone and moisturise as usual. Then do the following:
1 Smooth a light foundation or tinted moisturiser over your face and neck to even out skin colour.
2 If you have dark circles under your eyes, disguise them with a special concealer cream or fluid. It can also be used to cover spots.
3 Lightly and subtly apply a little blusher upwards along your cheekbones to define them and give your face more shape.
4 Make the most of your eyes — outline them with pencil or liner, smudging it slightly for a gentler effect. Fade it at the corners with a soft brush. If you wish to use eye shadow choose soft, muted shades for daywear — stronger shades are more suitable for evenings out. The shadow should fade upwards and outwards from the lids. Then colour your lashes with mascara to add thickness and glamour.
5 Coat your lips lightly with lipstick and pat with a tissue. The whole routine should take only 10 minutes. As you get more proficient, it will become second-nature and you will get even faster. For days on the beach, you may wish to simplify the process and wear only a good moisturising sunscreen, mascara and a pale lipstick.

You can change the shape of your eyes using clever make-up techniques with shadow, fading it inwards, outwards, upwards and below the eye.

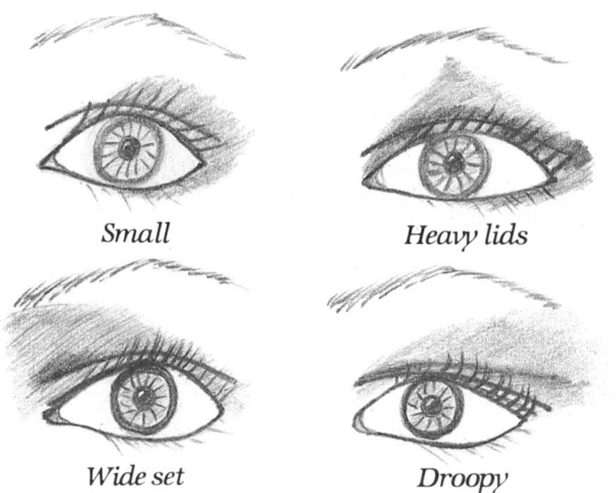

Make a point of avoiding fats in your diet

You should realise by now that you ought to eat less fat, especially saturated animal fats — cheese, butter, milk, cream, lard and fat on red meat. But how should you go about this and is there hidden fat in some of the products you tend to eat indiscriminately?
1 Opt for soft low-fat cheeses rather than high-fat hard cheeses like Cheddar. Of course, not all soft cheeses are low in fat, but you are quite safe with cottage cheese, fromage frais, ricotta and quark.
2 Make sure that the yoghurts you buy are low-fat varieties (and also unsweetened). Many yoghurts contain cream to give them a thicker, creamier texture.
3 Use skimmed milk in preference to full-fat milk, and give up cream. Try serving desserts with a topping of thick yoghurt instead.
4 Cook with vegetable oils rather than butter but use only a tiny amount. Don't deep-fry foods in lots of fat.
5 Beware of mayonnaise and sauces — many are high in fats, especially cream, oil and butter.
6 Eat good-quality nutritious wholemeal bread. If the bread tastes good you will automatically use less butter.
7 Don't add a pat of butter to cooked vegetables. Enjoy their true flavours and textures.

Khoshaf

100g/4oz mixed dried apricots, prunes or other dried fruit
grated rind and juice ½ lemon
good pinch cinnamon
15ml/1 tablespoon chopped almonds

Soak fruit in a little water overnight. Put in pan with soaking water and lemon juice and rind. Add cinnamon and bring to boil. Lower heat to simmer and cook until tender. Chill well and serve with almonds

Holiday tip

Order your foreign currency and travellers cheques now. Most banks require a few days notice so give your local branch enough time to get them in for you. If you forget, you can always change money at the bureau-de-change at the airport. Travellers cheques are very useful abroad — you can exchange them at most banks, or even pay with them directly in many hotels, restaurants and shops. Although you can buy them in many currencies, US dollars are best and widely accepted.

Learn the basics of good foot maintenance — give yourself a pedicure

Pay attention to your feet today. Are they the most neglected part of your body? Most women spend hours looking after their face, hair, hands and body and completely overlook their feet, yet they can cause you considerable pain and discomfort in years to come if you don't look after them now. Foot problems are commonplace — most are caused by ill-fitting shoes which are too small, too tight, too pointed, too narrow or too high. Callouses, corns, bunions, blisters, aching feet and legs and even back ache can result, so make sure that you are not a martyr to fashion and that you wear comfortable, flattish shoes. In summer and particularly on holiday, you can wear flat strappy sandals or even go barefoot to allow your feet to breathe more freely.

You should make daily washing a habit, either when you're in the bath or shower, or by soaking feet in a bowl of warm, soapy water. Use a pumice stone to rub away any dead skin. For tired, aching feet, try a tepid footbath of Epsom salts or add a few drops of lavender oil to the water. Afterwards, pat thoroughly dry taking care to dry well between the toes, and then dust with talcum powder. Once a week treat your feet to a complete pedicure:

1 Remove any old nail polish and then soak feet in warm water for about 10 minutes. Dry thoroughly.
2 Massage a little cuticle cream around the nails and gently ease back the cuticles with an orange stick, wrapped in cotton wool.
3 Trim your nails.
4 File your nails to smooth edges with a file or emery board.
5 Rub some moisturising cream into your feet.
6 Polish your nails in the usual way.
Do not skip this weekly routine. Feet are on show in summer and more noticeable than in the colder months when they are enclosed in boots and smart shoes. Look after your feet and they will reward you with graceful movement and good posture.

Your pedicure routine
1 *Soak feet in warm water or foot massager.*
2 *Rub cuticle cream into nails and ease back cuticles with orange stick.*
3 *Trim nails with clippers or nail scissors.*
4 *File nails smoothly with an emery board.*
5 *Moisturise feet all over with cream.*
6 *Separate toes with foam and polish nails.*

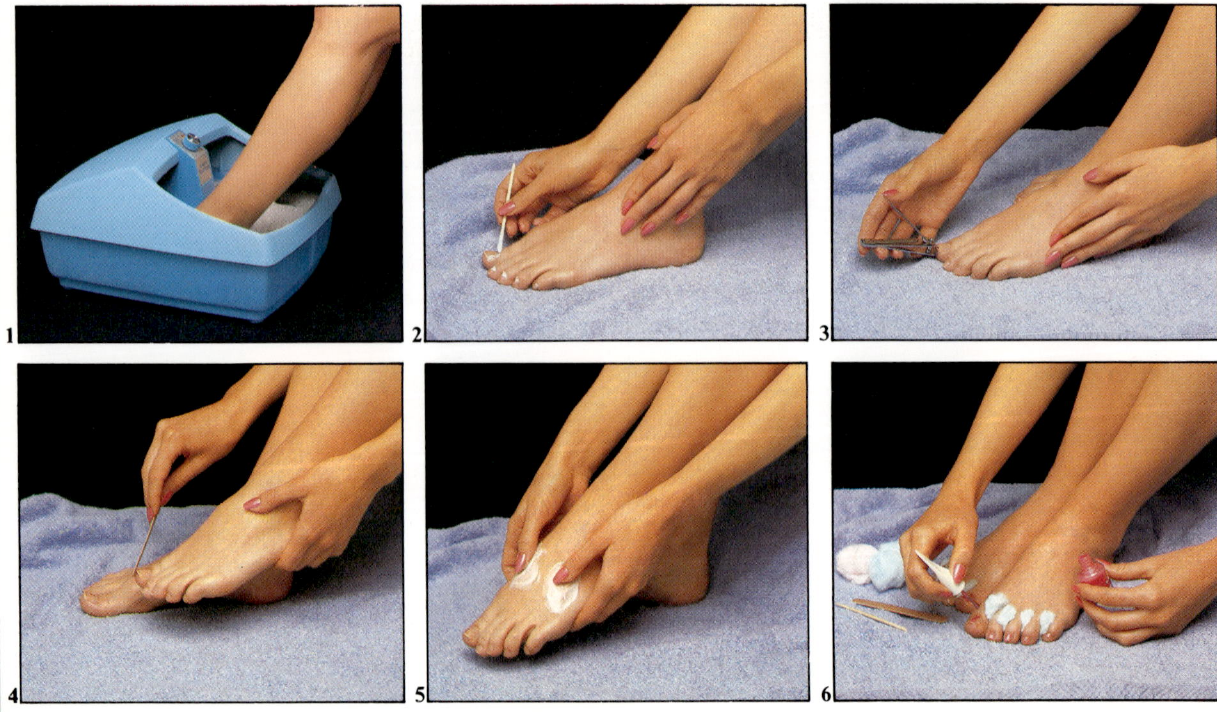

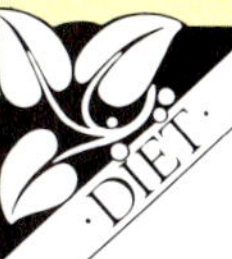

Weigh yourself and take note of the slimming tips

You have been on the diet and exercise programme for two weeks now so make a point of weighing yourself today and see if you have lost any weight since Day 1. If you think that the weight loss is disappointingly low, then take a look at yourself in a full-length mirror and reassess your new body shape. It will probably look a lot firmer and leaner. Are you managing to stick to the diet or do you have occasional lapses and inexplicable cravings for chocolate or French fries?

Here are a few hints which may help you to change your eating habits and slim more easily:

1 Don't eat lots of snacks — eat three filling meals instead. Use the guidelines laid down in the Diet Programme. Many snacks, such as sweets, chocolates, biscuits and crisps, are fattening and because of their high sugar or salt content you soon crave for more.
2 Throw left-overs away or freeze them. Do not put them in the fridge where you can nibble away at them.
3 Make a shopping list and stick to it when you go to the supermarket. Do not be tempted to try new convenience foods or to reach for the chocolates on display at the check-out. If you don't trust yourself, send someone out shopping for you with the list.
4 Enlist your family's help by giving them more healthy, slimming meals, too. It is difficult to stick to your diet if you are cooking beefburgers and chips for the kids.
5 Don't eat TV suppers and meals on trays. You will be more aware of what you eat and will feel more satisfied if you sit up at a table.

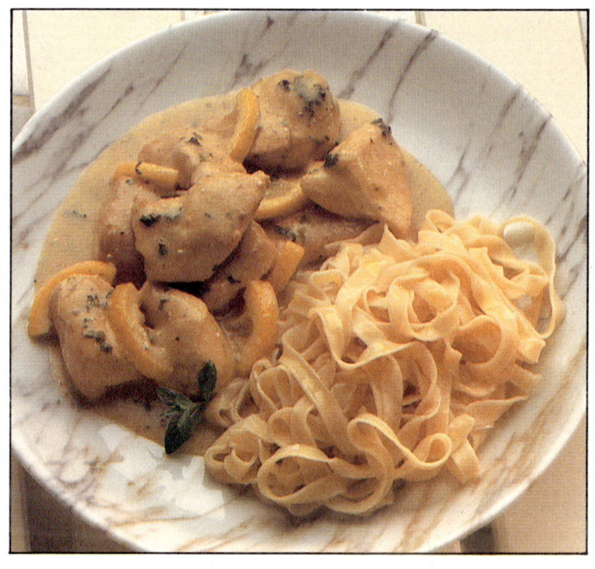

Lemon chicken

175g/6oz boned chicken breast in chunks
seasoned flour for dusting
10ml/2 teaspoons oil
75ml/3floz chicken stock
15ml/1 tablespoon dry sherry
5ml/1 teaspoon cornflour
75ml/3floz natural yoghurt
grated rind and juice of 1 lemon

Dust chicken with flour and sauté in oil until cooked. Bring stock and sherry to boil, blend cornflour with a little water and add to pan, stirring until thick over low heat. Add yoghurt and lemon. Heat through gently. Pour over chicken and serve with lemon.

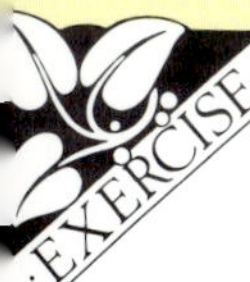

Go for a long walk and run up and down the stairs

Treat today as a kind of rest day and instead of indulging in some strenuous aerobic exercise, just go for a long walk. Walking is a good habit to encourage and you should do it whenever possible to burn up unwanted calories, increase stamina and get fit. Wear comfortable flat shoes which will give leg muscles a good work-out. Many women who are used to wearing high heels find flat shoes tiring at first and experience pain in their shins and calves. This is because their calf muscles are abnormally short and need stretching out. If this is the case with you, then try doing some of the calf stretches before you walk, run or jog. Gradually increase your speed and the distance covered. If you want to look slimmer and leaner, you will have to walk more briskly. A leisurely amble round the shops will have little if any benefit. Also, try to include some hillwork in your walks — choose a route which is not on the level but includes some sharp inclines to make you work harder. Walk for at least 30-45 minutes.

After your walk, do some stair-climbing. Aim for 100-150 steps as fast as you can go. This may mean climbing up several flights in a block of flats or offices, or running up and down the same staircase at home. Aim for a time of about three minutes, and repeat three times during the day. This is one of the best ways of burning up calories fast and getting slim.

Day 19

Give yourself a regular monthly breast-check

If you want beautiful breasts, you cannot leave them to their own devices. You can improve their tone and firm up the supporting muscles with regular swimming and special exercises. These are particularly important if you have had a baby recently.
1 Stand with your elbows at shoulder height, palms of your hands pressed together. Press as hard as you can, hold for a count of five and then relax. Repeat 10 times.
2 Stand with your arms by your sides. Now swing your arms out forwards and then back over your shoulders in big circles. Make 10 circles and repeat the other way.
When exercising always wear a good supporting bra. Most companies now make special sports bras which are light and comfortable, made of cotton and give your bust the additional support it needs when running or working-out. To prevent stretch marks on your breasts, especially during pregnancy, gently rub in some moisturising cream and make sure you eat plenty of vitamin-E rich foods or take it in supplement form daily. Zinc is another important nutrient. Your Diet Programme will provide your daily requirements but if you have stretch marks, take a supplement as well.

All women should regularly check their breasts to detect any lumps or changes. The best time is every month after your period. Stand in front of a mirror, undressed to the waist and raise your arms above your head and then lower them to your hips. Look at the shape of your breasts and how they hang. They should be firm and well-shaped. Now lift your left breast with your left hand and gently examine it, especially in the area between the nipple and your armpit, feeling carefully for any lumps or thickening. It is best to do this lying down. Repeat the exercise with the other breast. If your breasts are sore, there is any abnormal discharge or lumpiness, consult your doctor right away. Over 90 per cent of lumps are benign (not cancerous), but it is just as well to be on the safe side.

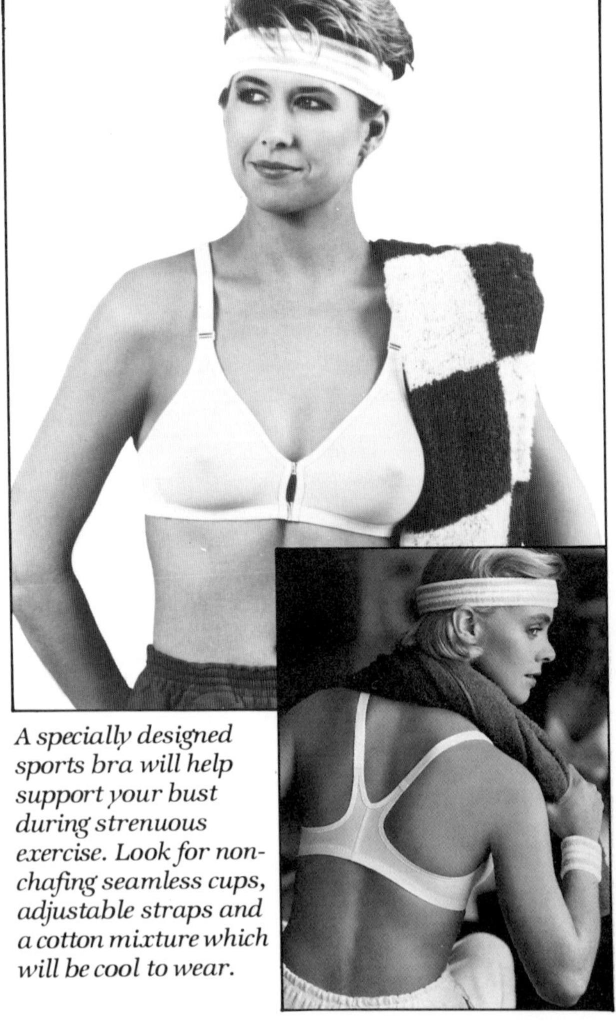

A specially designed sports bra will help support your bust during strenuous exercise. Look for non-chafing seamless cups, adjustable straps and a cotton mixture which will be cool to wear.

Holiday tip

Check your luggage for faulty locks, broken handles and straps, missing keys and damaged zips. You still have time to get it repaired or buy replacements if necessary. Don't take chances with damaged luggage — even though you may tape it up and secure it with large rolls of string, it may still burst open in transit and spill your clothes across the customs hall. If you need luggage wheels, an extra strap or lightweight shoulder bag, now is the time to buy them.

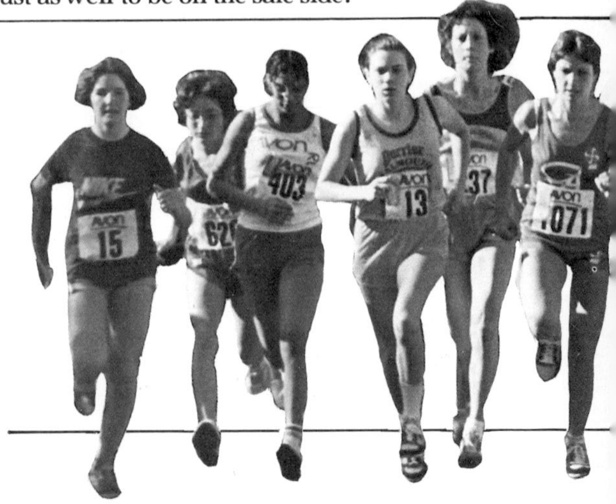

DIET

Take zinc every day for beauty and health

One of the most overlooked nutrients is zinc, yet this mineral can have far-reaching physical and beauty benefits. Zinc makes your skin more supple, less prone to stretch marks and it is essential for growth. If you are deficient in zinc, you are likely to get depressed, have mood swings and even damage your sense of taste. If you want beautiful skin and hair and healthy nails without white spots, you need more zinc. Although it is found in lots of foods — seafoods, nuts, meat, whole grain bread and green vegetables — it may be difficult to eat in sufficient quantities, mostly due to processing and poor diet. White bread has only 25 per cent of the zinc of wholemeal bread; white sugar has no zinc; and many green vegetables lose their zinc if sprayed with 'NPK' fertilisers. Women are in particular need of zinc, especially if they take a contraceptive pill or crash-diet regularly. If this applies to you, then make sure you take a daily zinc supplement of, say, 15-20 mg.

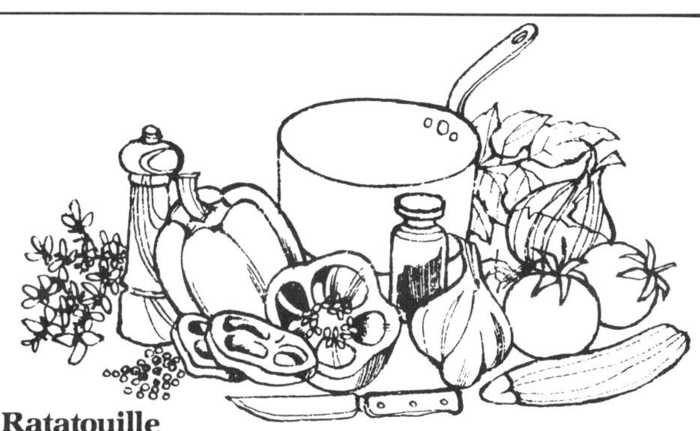

Ratatouille

1 small onion, sliced
½ green pepper, sliced
½ red pepper, sliced
1 clove garlic, crushed
1 courgette, sliced
5ml/1 teaspoon olive oil
2 tomatoes, skinned and chopped
fresh herbs eg. chopped basil, oregano
few coriander seeds, crushed
salt and pepper

Sauté onion, peppers, garlic and courgette in oil until soft. Add tomato and cook gently for 10-15 minutes until thick and tender. Add coriander and seasoning. Serve hot or cold.

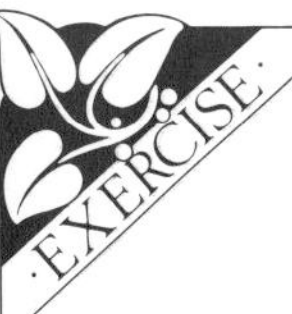

EXERCISE

Go running to get aerobically fit and strong

It's another jogging day today so get changed and warmed-up and then set out for a 20 minute run interspersed with walking whenever necessary. You will probably find that although the going is tough at first, after about 10 minutes or so you will experience what is known in the running fraternity as 'your second wind'. Suddenly, you will breathe more easily and you will seem to flow better as you run along. After the initial hard work and effort it will all seem worthwhile and enjoyable. If you enjoy running and want to keep it up in the future it may be worth your while to join a local jogging or athletics club. Most clubs welcome beginners and will offer support and advice. Get hold of some running and fitness magazines — they often have a club directory.

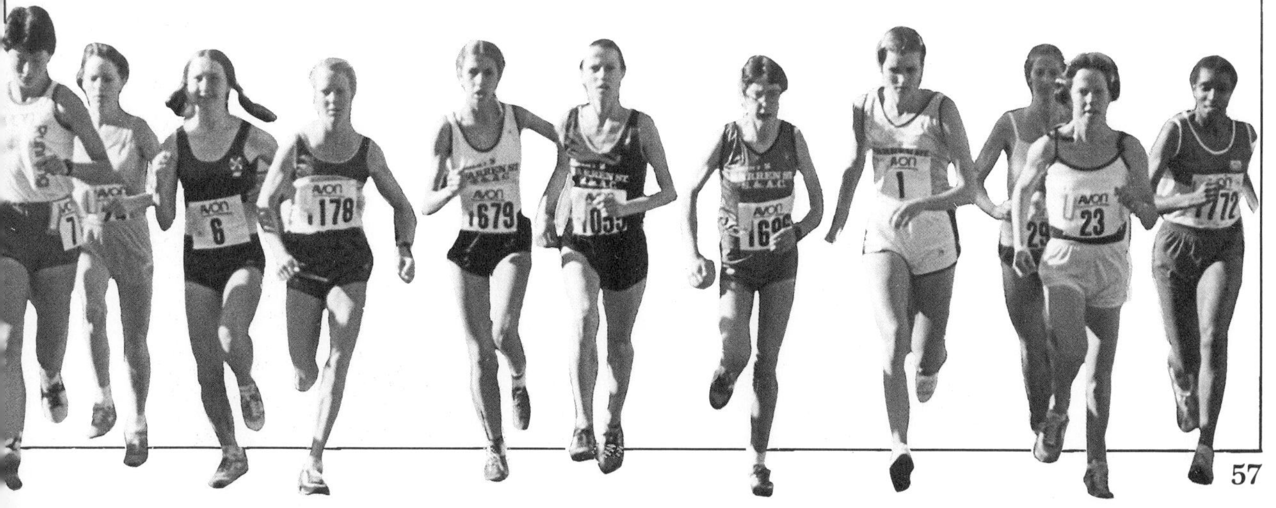

Day 20

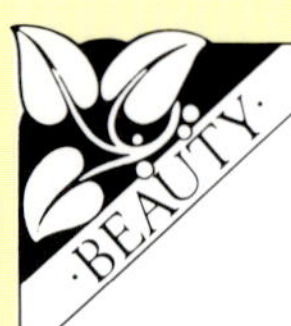

Beauty treatments, diet and exercise for lovely legs

Legs have to look extra-good on holiday so start taking care of them now. Begin by removing any hair. You can shave it off with a wet razor and plenty of foam, or a dry electric razor. Shaving is the quickest and easiest method of hair removal but it does result in stubbly regrowth. A depilatory cream is more messy but will leave legs silky smooth. Or you can wax them for long-lasting results, either with a do-it-yourself kit at home or at a beauty salon.

If your knees are rough-looking with coarse, dry skin, then rub them with soap to work up a rich lather and then attack with a massage glove to remove any dead skin. Add a little oil to the bath water and moisturise them after drying. Any unsightly patches of cellulite on your upper thighs can also be broken down with deep massage (see Day 7 on page 28) and good diet.

Check your legs for tiny broken veins — although there is virtually no cure for these, you can avoid them in future by eating plenty of citrus fruits and other vitamin C-rich foods. A healthy diet will also help prevent varicose veins — your legs' worst enemies. Constipation and overweight are common causes, especially during pregnancy, so make sure you eat lots of high-fibre foods (fruit, vegetables, whole grain bread and cereals). Regular exercise will improve the circulation in your legs and tone up muscles to make them more shapely. Other ways of avoiding varicose veins include: taking daily supplements of vitamin E, not standing still for long periods, putting feet up level with your hips when resting, and not sitting for long with your legs crossed.

If your legs are really pale when it's too hot to wear stockings and you haven't the time or the sunshine to build up a tan, use a sunlamp or a fake tanning lotion to give them a healthy-looking colour. It gives you a headstart on your holiday.

Beautiful legs are a great asset to any woman. Keep your legs smooth with waxing or hair removal. Add oil to your bathwater to counteract dry skin and moisturise regularly. Massage and friction improve circulation, prevent little broken veins on the surface of the skin, and break down any stubborn patches of ugly cellulite.

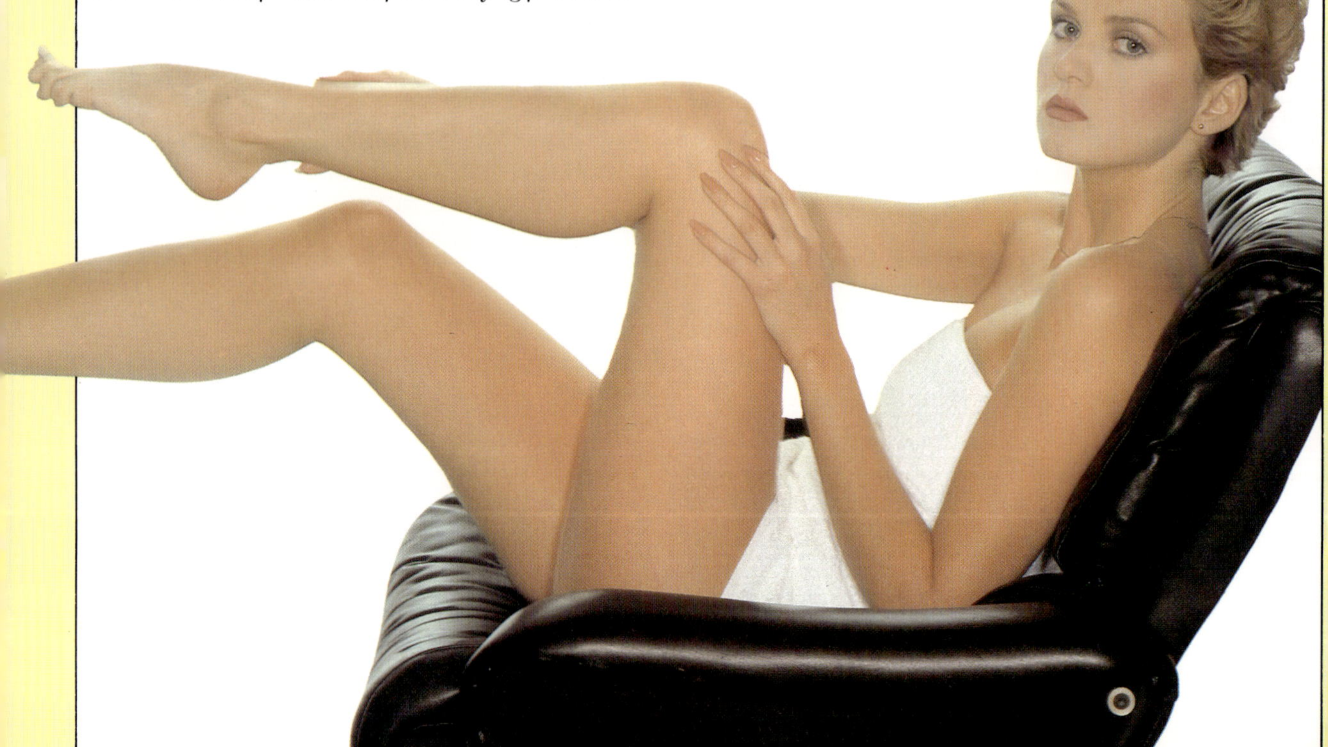

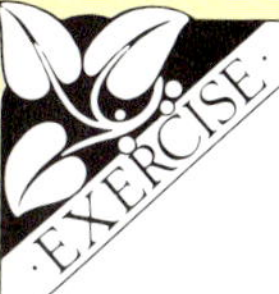

Exercise on court with a game of tennis

For a complete change, why not book a tennis court for a game later today. All you need are a partner, tennis racket, tennis shoes and a set of balls. Then you can knock-up and have a game. Aim to play for at least an hour and try to make each other run about the court as much as possible. If the weather's bad and only outdoor courts are available, have a game of squash or badminton instead. Most sports centres and clubs have their own facilities and you can hire them out for an hour. Remember to stretch and warm-up first to help protect you against injury.

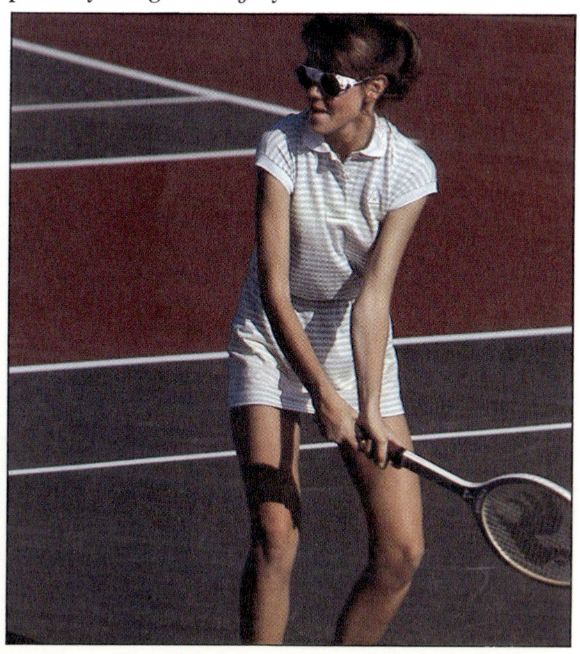

Holiday tip

Check your summer wardrobe to see if any clothes you plan to take on holiday need cleaning or repairing. Look for broken zips, missing buttons and loose hems. Put them right now rather than leave them to the last minute on the eve of your departure. Have you got enough cool summer dresses, evening wear, bikinis and swimsuits? Even though you can wash them out and hang them up to dry above the bath or on the hotel balcony, you will need several changes of beach clothes. Go on a shopping trip and treat yourself to some new clothes.

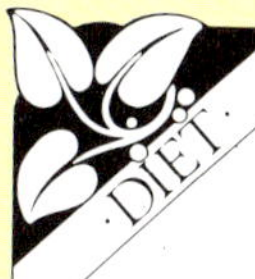

Grow your own herbs for health and beauty

Why not grow your own herb garden for flavouring meals and instant beauty treatments? Fresh herbs are an excellent source of vitamins and minerals and at the end of the summer you can dry them for using throughout the winter. You do not need a large piece of land — a window box, patio tubs or a sunny kitchen windowsill lined with pots will do. Most herbs grow well in pots, even small trees like bay. They need sunshine and light, fertile soil. You can buy small plants or grow them from seed yourself in late spring and early summer. Choose from the following: balm, basil, bay, chervil, chives, marjoram, mint, oregano, parsley, rosemary, sage, tarragon and thyme. They will all look pretty and will fill the house and garden with their beautiful fragrance.

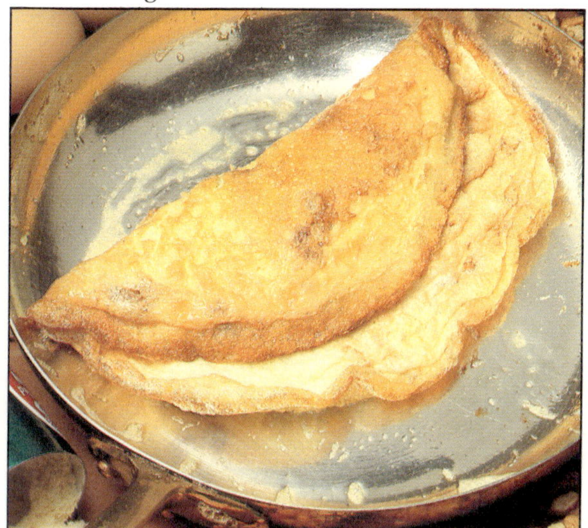

Cheese and walnut omelette

2 eggs
10ml/2 teaspoons water
salt and pepper
small knob butter
25g/1oz Parmesan cheese, grated
25g/1oz walnuts, chopped

Beat the eggs with the water and seasoning lightly with a fork. Melt the butter in a non-stick omelette pan and pour in the egg mixture. Cook over gentle heat, drawing in the runny mixture from the sides. Add the cheese and nuts and cook until set and golden underneath. Fold over and serve with salad.

Day 21

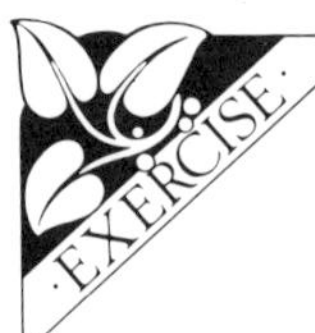

Try room-running if you haven't the time to go out

Choose between jogging, swimming or cycling today and aim to increase your distance slightly and the time you spend exercising. It is worth bearing in mind that if you can't get out for some reason, you can always try room-running on the spot. This form of home aerobics will exercise your heart and help maintain your newly acquired level of fitness. When you jog on the spot, try raising your knees as high as you can to work your body even harder. Start off by running in place for three minutes, then walk on the spot for one minute, run for another three minutes and walk for one minute.

If you find this too boring, you could try working-out or doing some running around the largest room in the house with weights — either the sort you hold or the strap-around wristlet kind. Both are available from good sporting goods stores. Weights make muscles work harder so that they become even stronger and firmer. As long as you use only 1kg/2lb weights and perform the exercises with plenty of repetitions, you will not put on muscle bulk. It is practically impossible for women to do so, anyway. You can also purchase strap-on ankle weights which fit snugly round your legs and make leg strengthening exercises more efficient — ideal for slimming down heavy ankles and thighs and firming up long-unused muscles. So if you want a shapely body, go out and buy some weights and don't worry about not being feminine.

These people are working-out with weights at London's Big Apple Health Studios.

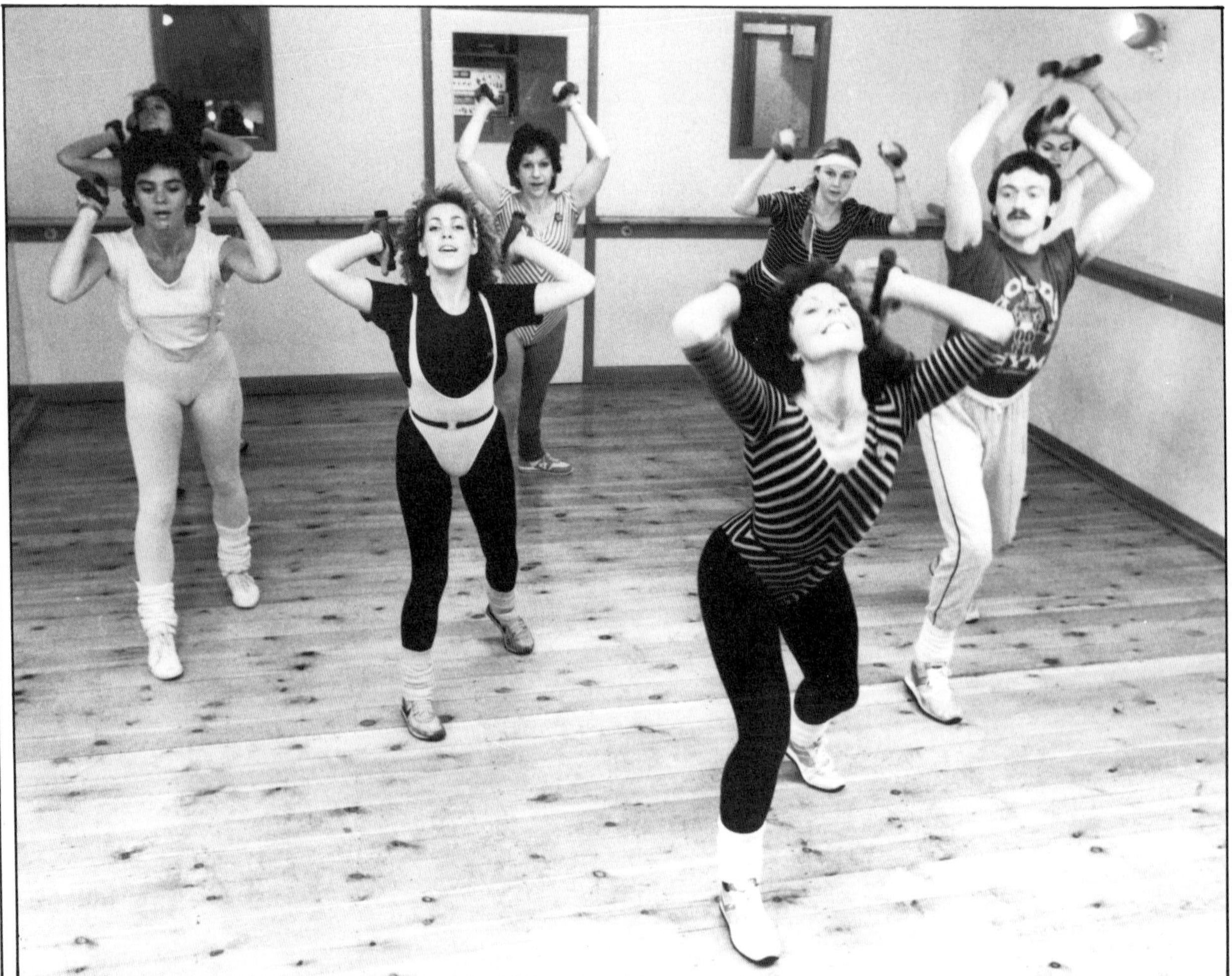

Spring-clean your body with gentle skin-brushing

Another way of attacking cellulite and speeding up the loss of toxic wastes through your skin is a technique called skin brushing. For this you will need a rough hemp massage mit or a bristle brush with a long handle. Unlike most forms of massage and friction, skin brushing should be done before, not after, a bath or shower when your skin is really dry.

1 Starting with your feet, brush gently but firmly up your legs on both sides.

2 With sweeping strokes, continue brushing up your body — your stomach, chest and neck.

3 Then work upwards from your hands along your arms to the shoulders and across the back of your neck.

Skin brushing will increase your blood circulation, especially in areas where cellulite is concentrated. Afterwards, have a warm bath or shower and finish off with a cold shower to leave you really tingling all over.

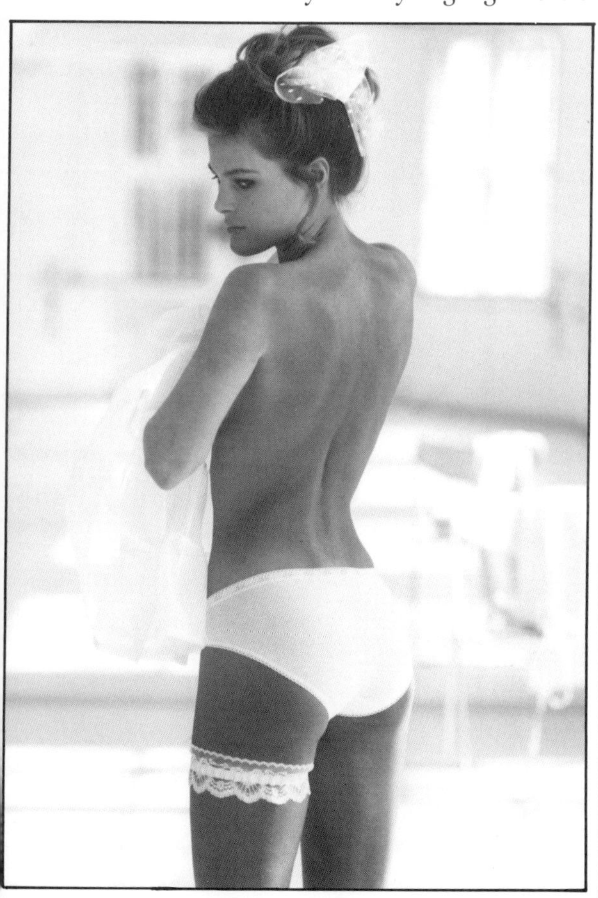

·DIET·

Grow your own fruit and vegetables the natural organic way

If you want to eat a truly healthy diet, you must either buy organically grown fruit and vegetables or, better still, grow your own. These are fresh produce which have not been treated with chemical sprays and fertilisers. They are grown in healthy, organic soil using only compost as a fertiliser to enrich the soil. Pests are controlled with organic sprays such as derris. You need only a small plot of ground to grow a surprisingly large crop of vegetables. If you live in an apartment, you might consider getting an allotment from your local authority. Gardening is a pleasant way to spend your free time, and good exercise, too. In this way, you can control your environment yourself and know exactly what goes into the food you eat. Plant some fruit trees and bushes for summer and autumn harvesting, and freeze all the fruit and vegetables you cannot eat immediately for the long winter months.

Chilled cucumber soup

1 spring onion, chopped
⅓ cucumber, peeled and diced
150ml/¼ pint natural yoghurt
juice of ½ small lemon
15ml/1 tablespoon fresh mint
dash wine vinegar
salt and pepper
3 coriander seeds (optional)

Blend all ingredients until smooth. Chill before eating. Serve garnished with additional chopped herbs if wished.

Holiday tip

Remember to cancel the milk and newspapers before you leave for your holiday. Do it discreetly so that only people you trust will know that the house is going to be empty. You can also tell the local police and give them an address or telephone number where you can be contacted in case of emergencies. Deposit anything valuable in the bank — don't attempt to stash it away under a mattress, floorboards or in the cellar. Burglars look *everywhere.*

Holiday make-up

Look stunning on the beach this summer by keeping make-up to a minimum. The look to aim for is light and healthy-looking — perfect for showing off your tan and giving your skin a breather. Here's how to achieve your best beach looks and get a healthy summer glow.

Skin — keep the moisture in

Your skin needs extra protection from the sun, sea and wind so always wear a good moisturiser to guard against drying and flaking. A light tinted moisturiser with its own built-in sunscreen is a good idea for giving protection as well as colour. Heavier make-ups and foundations tend to run and go streaky in hot weather and should be avoided. By wearing the minimum of make-up, you are allowing your skin to breathe and renew itself. If you prefer not to use make-up at all, opt for a deep-action moisturiser and a little translucent powder or a light gel to add summer shine.

For evenings out, you can wear a pretty bronze tinted gel or gloss which will make the most of your tan. A hint of blusher, skilfully applied, can define your cheekbones and add subtle highlights.

Don't forget the rest of your body — moisturise mornings and evenings with cocoa butter or another tropically scented natural moisturiser. Remember that although it is great to escape from city pollution to fresh sea air and sunshine, skin still needs looking after and adequate protection.

Eyes — shade them from the sun

Eye make-up can soon look streaked and messy in the sea and on the beach so wear waterproof shadow and mascara or, better still, dye your eyelashes black, brown or blue. You can do this yourself at home or visit a beauty salon. Tinted lashes look longer and thicker and help emphasise your eyes.

After a day on the beach, try refreshing tired eyes with cooling cotton wool pads soaked in witch hazel. Or squeeze out a couple of cold tea bags and place them over your eyes for 10 minutes. Lie down and rest, and you will feel invigorated and ready to face the evening.

Never risk your eyes in the sun, so make sure that you have a pair of quality sunglasses to protect them from glare, bright sunlight and eyestrain. The best ones are dark enough to absorb 75 to 90 per cent of sunlight, and a good rule of thumb when choosing sunglasses is that if you can see your eyes through the lenses they are not sufficiently dark. Go for neutral colours like grey, brown and sage-green as these are most effective at absorbing light. They also transmit the colour spectrum without distortion so there is no danger of getting a headache as with some cheaper shades.

Photochromatic lenses are very popular at the moment but most transmit about 45 per cent of light and although they often look very flattering, they may not be suitable for dazzling sunlight. Choose lenses which are coated or polarised — mirror-coated ones are particularly good as they reflect heat and are cool to wear. Remember also that shatterproof safety glass is often better than plastic lenses which scratch easily.

There is such a wide range of fashionable sunglasses with good lenses and colourful frames that you shouldn't have any trouble finding a pair that will flatter your face and match your wardrobe.

Hands and feet — basic sun maintenance

These are more visible in summer so make sure you look after them properly. Nothing looks worse than dirty, cracked nails with flaking nail varnish. Give them a regular manicure and pedicure and then apply a coat of pretty pearly pink or clear varnish. Hands and feet have a hard time in sunshine, chlorinated pools and sea-water so rub in plenty of moisturising cream and always wear a sunscreen on the beach.

Lips — don't just gloss over them

Lips need special protection in the sun to prevent burning and blisters. Apply a sunscreen in a handy swivel case or one of the protective lip glosses with a built-in sunblock. Because they contain no oils or protective melanin, lips are in a high-risk burning category so don't forget to cover them with a special screen *before* setting out for the beach and to reapply it throughout the day, especially after swimming.

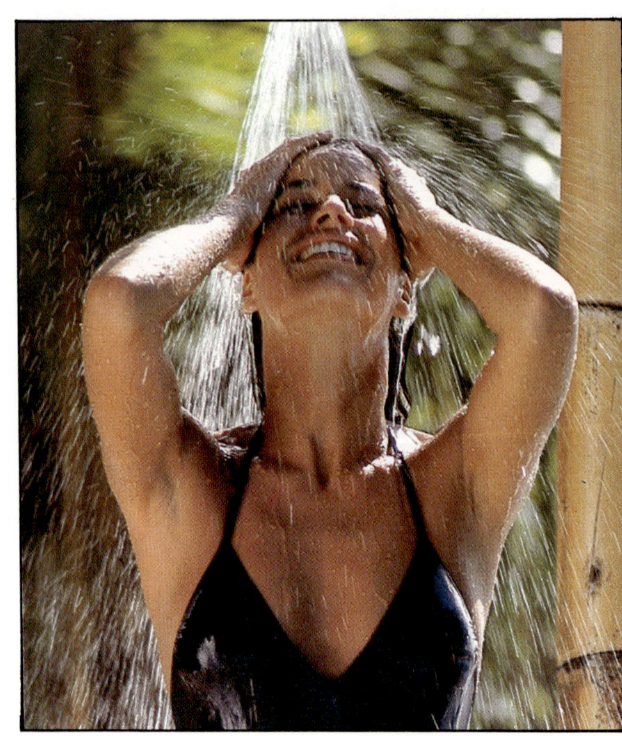

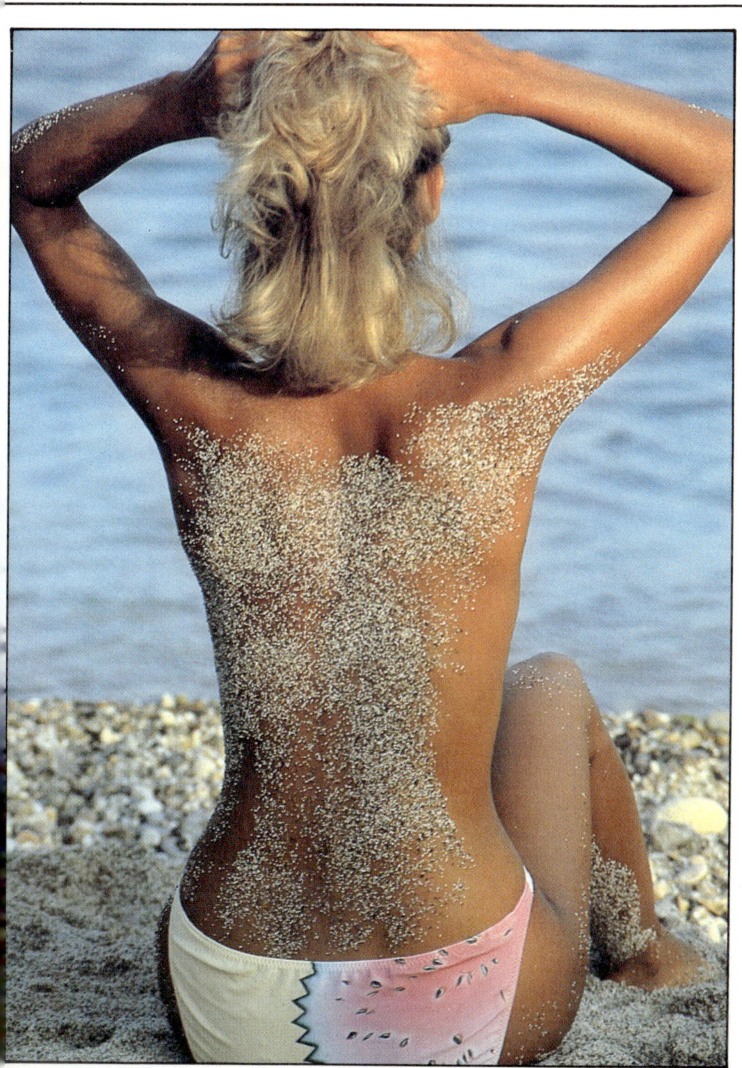

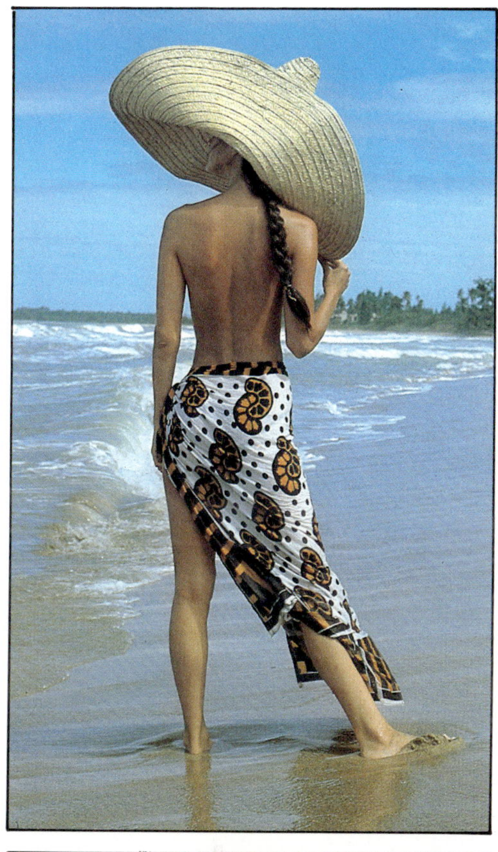

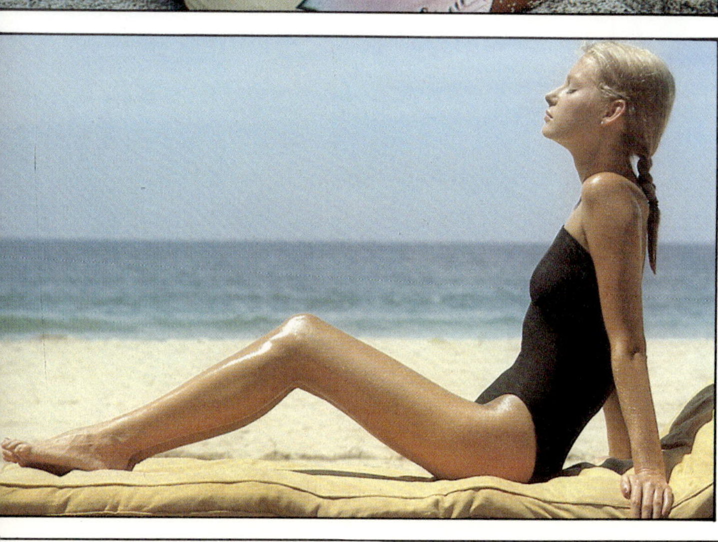

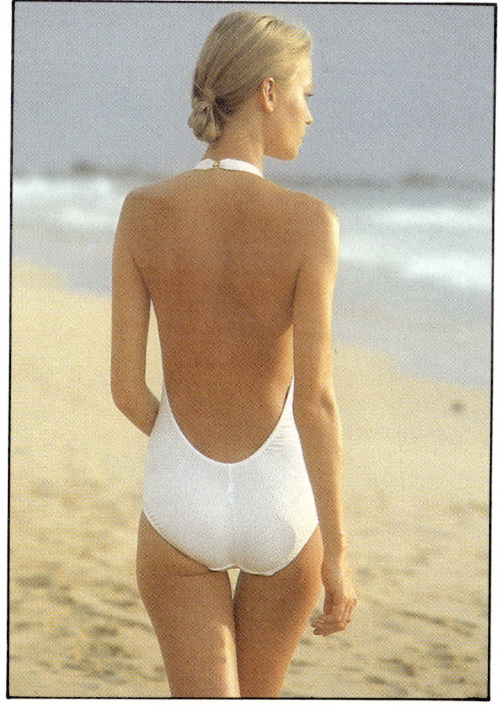

Give your scalp a massage and colour your hair

Massaging your scalp increases circulation and boosts hair growth. It also helps hair grow thicker and stronger. Don't worry that you might make greasy hair more oily by over-stimulating the follicles — you won't. On the contrary, massage tends to normalise an over-oily condition and may cure all your hair problems.

To massage your scalp, use the fingertips and palms of your hands and work upwards and inwards from the sides of your head in small circular movements. Your scalp, not your fingers, should be moving. Gradually work up to the top of your head and then to the front and back. You can do this massage every day as there is no need to do it on wet hair. If you wish to wash your hair today, however, massage your scalp first and think about changing your hair colour — not drastically but subtly to add highlights and gloss to dull hair. Use a temporary colourant or one of the more natural vegetable alternatives — camomile for blondes or henna for brunettes and raven black hair to give it a reddish glow. Even if you are just fair or a mousy light brown, you can achieve a lovely streaked effect with a camomile rinse, using dried camomile flowers, water and a little lemon juice. Bring the water to the boil, then simmer the flowers for 10-15 minutes. Strain, cool, rinse and towel-dry.

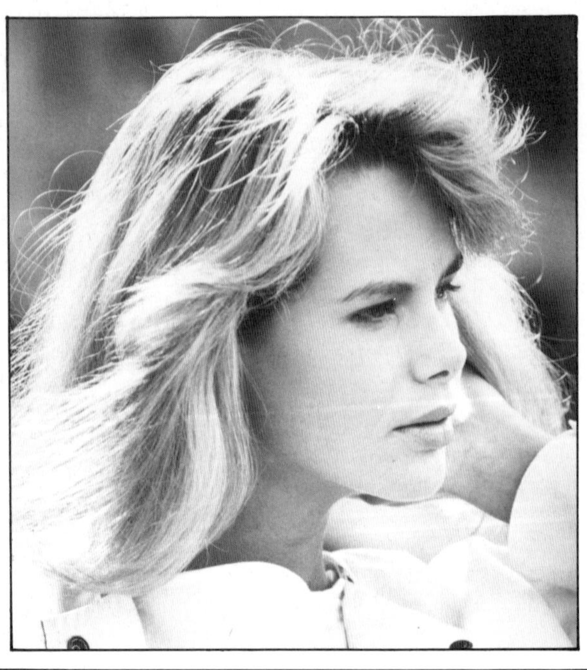

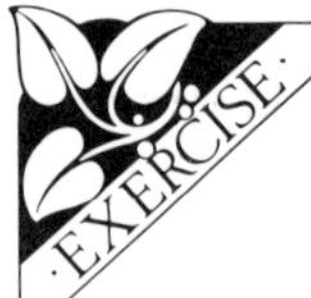

How to avoid common running aches and pains

It's another jogging session today so follow your usual routine. By now, you shouldn't need any reminding about the importance of warming-up first, stretching and cooling-down after your run. It is a good idea to know how to treat some of the common aches and pains experienced by runners. Avoid chafing under your arms by applying some petroleum jelly before you set out. You can use this to prevent blisters on your feet if you dislike wearing socks. If you get muscle soreness or swelling in your legs, put an ice pack on the area for 10 minutes when you get back from your run. You can buy handy slim packs to keep in the freezer or just use a polythene bag filled with ice cubes. Always put a layer of cloth between the ice and your skin to prevent burning. If you get stitch in your side when out running, slow down and try to jog through it, using deep breathing to ease out any pain. Any injuries that persist should be referred to a physiotherapist or doctor for professional treatment. Some hospitals now run special sports clinics which offer advice and specialist treatment. Most doctors tend to know little about athletic injuries and counsel you to stop running if you complain that your legs/back/feet hurt but only when you run! If this is your experience, find another more sympathetic doctor or visit a qualified physiotherapist.

It is important to choose a running shoe with the right sole as shown below. A wavy, flat sole is ideal for road-running but slippery on grass. A waffle sole with studs is perfect for rough ground and muddy paths. A cantilever sole gives good shock absorption and helps protect you against injury.

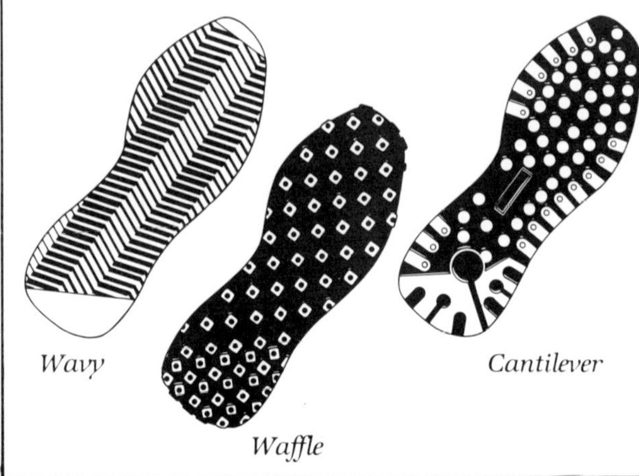

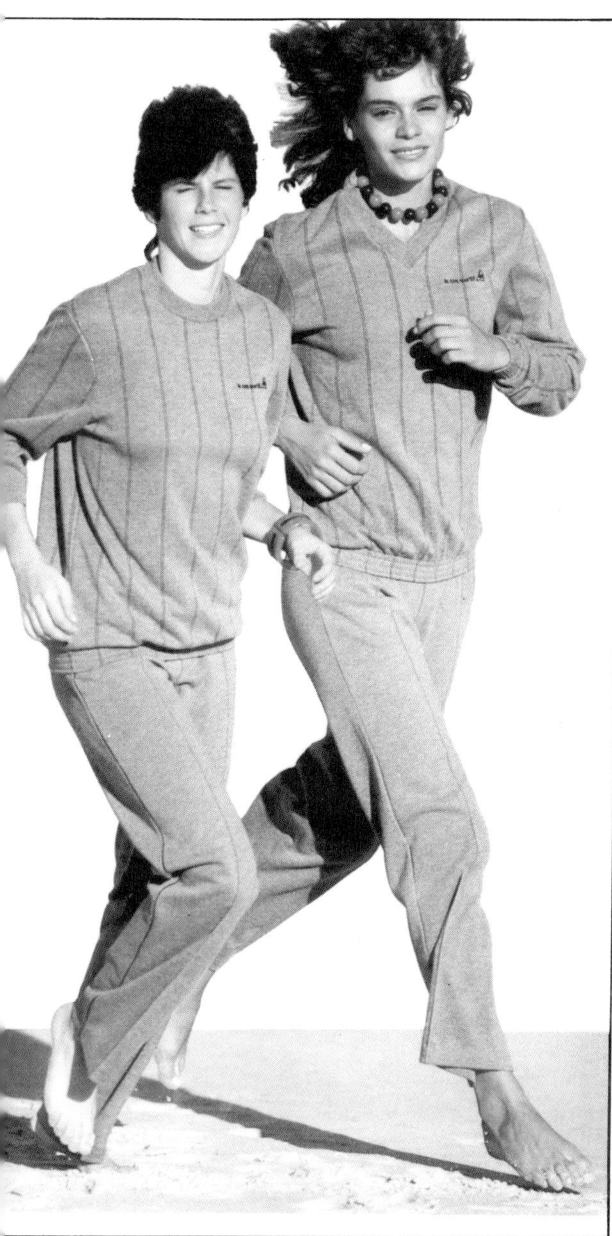

Holiday tip

Prepare to shade yourself from the hot sun on holiday. A beach umbrella does not offer full protection as it allows about 50 per cent of ultra-violet rays to penetrate through to you. A sun hat will help protect your head and guard against sunstroke so buy one now if you haven't already got one. Remember also that while a dry T-shirt gives maximum protection, a wet one acts as a filter for up to 40 per cent of burning rays.

Test for sensitive reactions to certain foods

An increasing number of people are finding that they are sensitive to certain foods, especially wheat products, milk and dairy foods, and processed foods which contain additives, especially monosodium glutamate, red food colouring and certain preservatives. Craving for sweet foods and an insatiable appetite, nervousness, mood swings, rashes, eczema and hyperactivity may be related to food allergies. If you think that your diet may be the culprit, then stick to the fresh whole foods diet programme and see if the condition improves. If you suspect a certain food in your diet, try leaving it out for a week or so and see if you feel better. If eliminating processed and dairy foods, cheese, white sugar and flour have no effect, you can always go along to an allergy clinic and be tested for sensitive reactions to foods

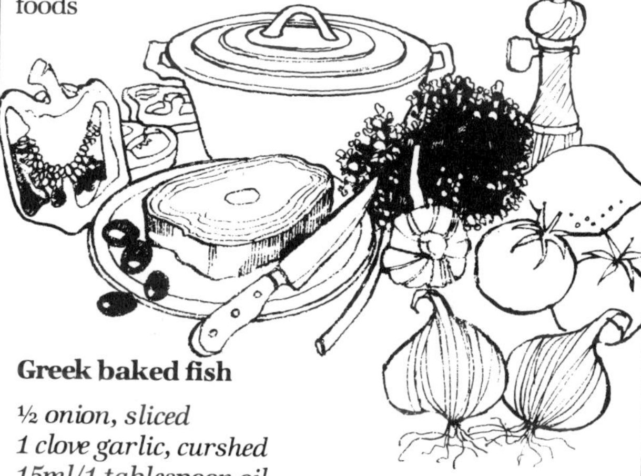

Greek baked fish

½ onion, sliced
1 clove garlic, curshed
15ml/1 tablespoon oil
100ml/4floz water
juice of ½ lemon
strip lemon rind
1 cod or halibut steak
1 large tomato, skinned and sliced
3 slices red or green pepper
4 black olives
salt and pepper
chopped parsley

Sauté onion and garlic in oil until soft. Add water, lemon juice and rind. Bring to boil. Cover and simmer for 15 minutes. Put fish in ovenproof dish. Cover with tomato and pepper slices. Pour over the onion mixture and dot with olives. Season and bake in preheated oven at 190°/375°F/gas 5 for 20 minutes. Garnish with parsley and serve.

Day 23

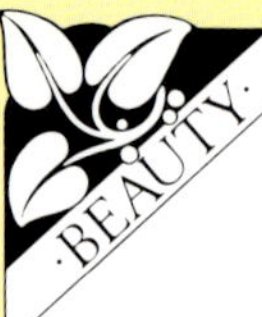

Condition and nourish your skin with masks and creams

Treat yourself to a deep action face mask today to revitalise, condition and stimulate your skin. After removing it and rinsing clean, check your skin in a magnifying mirror and compare it with the way it was at the beginning of the Programme. Is it softer, more translucent, less blemished and clearer? It should be if you have been sticking to the diet and performing your daily cleansing, toning and moisturising routine. If it still needs extra attention, try using a nourishing night cream before going to bed. Apply lightly — you don't have to paste it on thickly as your skin can only absorb a little. A regular facial at a beauty salon may help revive tired skin — modern cathiodermie and ozone treatments often prove helpful.

A facial (1) and cathiodermie treatment (2) are two luxurious ways to revive skin, and will leave it feeling smooth, moist and wonderfully refreshed. Treat yourself today at a beauty salon.

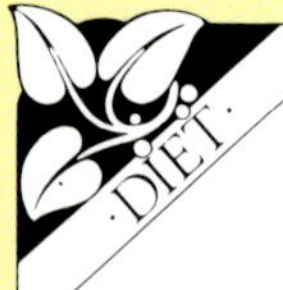

An apple a day keeps the doctor away

So the old adage goes and scientists are now proving that there may be some truth in it. Apples make quick, refreshing snacks, providing us with energy and fibre. They are low in calories and provide vitamins and minerals, too. They also play an important part in cleaning teeth and helping to keep them strong and healthy. Apples come in a wide range of delicious flavours — from the green granny smiths and golden delicious to deep red Johnathans and golden russets, rosy tinged sturmers and blushing Coxes. Carry an apple around with you — to work, your exercise class, on walks and shopping trips. Its natural fibre content makes it a filling, healthy fast food which will fight off hunger pangs. You can also use it in salads, desserts (with yoghurt) and even as a filling for omelettes chopped up with creamy blue cheese, or cottage cheese and herbs.

1

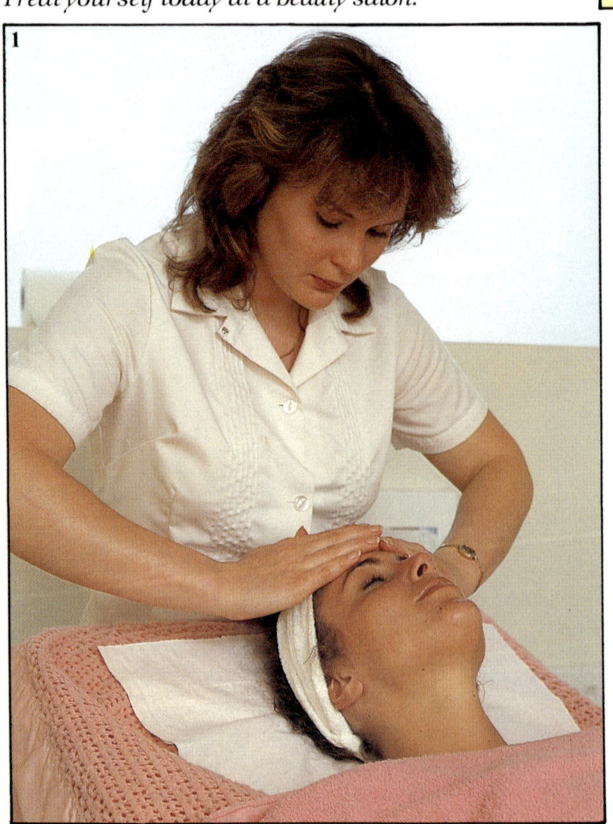

2

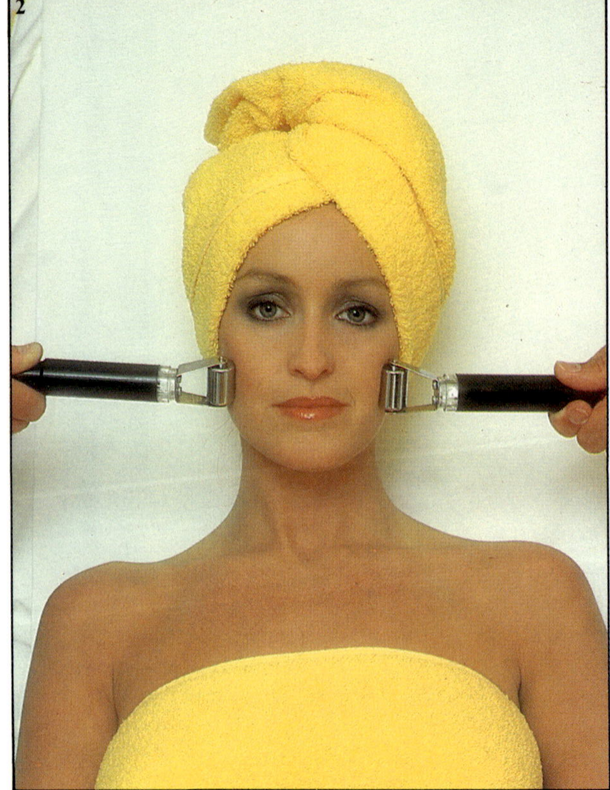

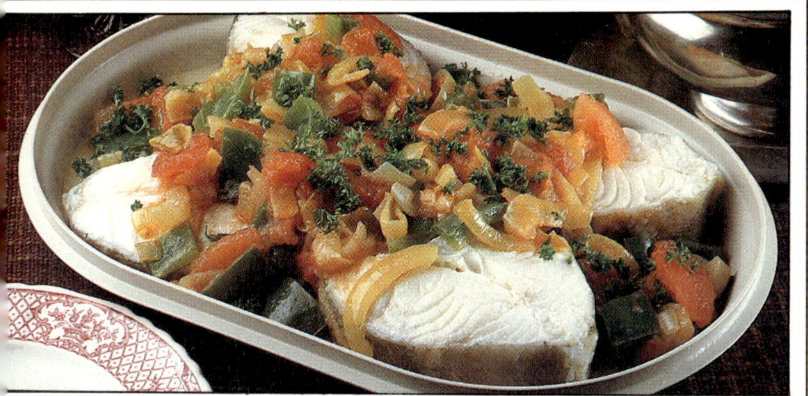

Mediterranean fish

1 cod or halibut steak
oil
½ small onion, chopped
1 tomato, skinned and chopped
¼ green pepper, diced
salt and pepper
100ml/4 floz fish stock or white wine
chopped parsley

Place the fish steak or cutlet in a well-oiled baking dish. Top with the onion, tomato, green pepper and season well. Pour in the stock or wine and cover with a lid. Bake in a moderate oven at 180°C, 350°F, gas 4 for about 20 minutes, or until the fish is cooked and tender. Sprinkle with plenty of chopped fresh parsley.

Holiday tip

Let your neighbours know that you are taking a holiday soon. They may be kind enough to water your house-plants and garden for you while you're away. Leave a set of keys with them if they are good friends in case of emergencies or if you would like them to pop in and put on a light in the evenings to deter would-be burglars. Ask them to keep an eye out for strangers near the house or to feed the cat if you have one. Fit a special cat door or send kitty for a holiday at the local cattery.

EXERCISE

Make your work-out harder with more repetitions

Run through your work-out today, incorporating all the exercises you have learnt to date. In this way, you will work every area of your body. You should be feeling firmer and stronger than you did when you started, and looking slimmer, too. You can make your work-out harder and more strenuous by increasing the repetitions of different exercises. For instance, if you find 10 sit-ups are easy, do 15 or even 20 instead. You may like to consider joining a California stretch or aerobic class, perhaps even an intermediate or advanced one depending on how fit and strong you are feeling. It's fun to exercise with other people, especially if you lack the self-discipline to work-out regularly at home by yourself. Then you can continue with your exercises long after the Programme has finished.

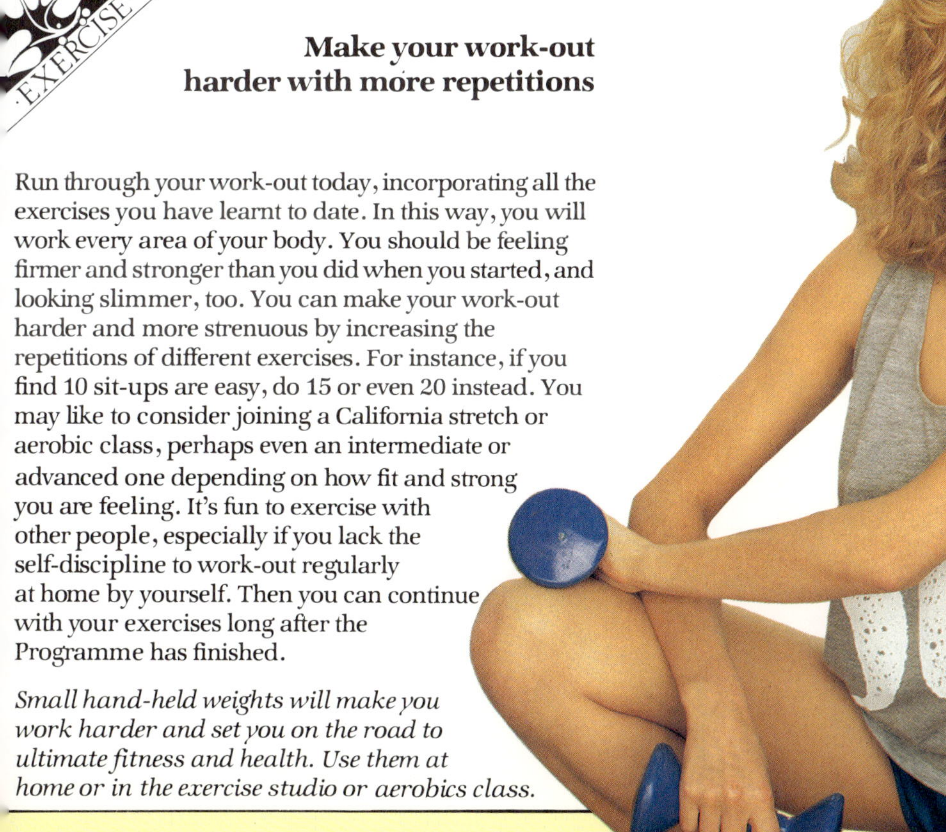

Small hand-held weights will make you work harder and set you on the road to ultimate fitness and health. Use them at home or in the exercise studio or aerobics class.

Day 24

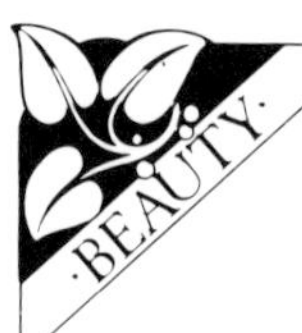

Use wax for keeping legs smooth and beautiful

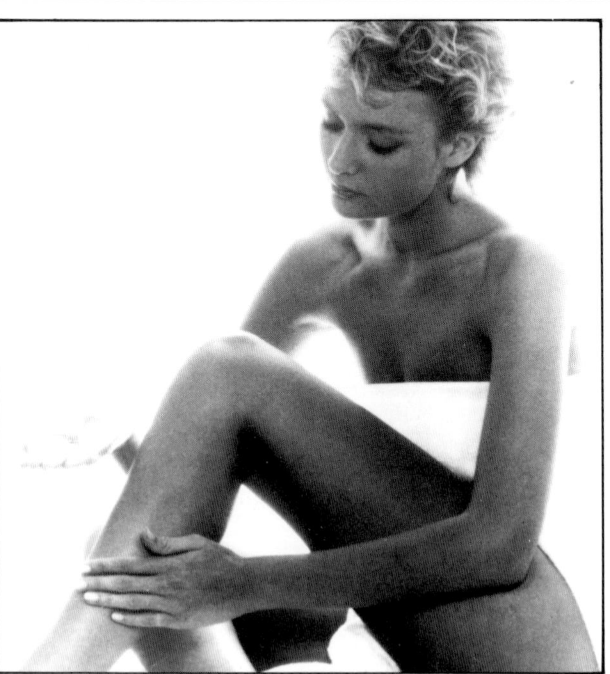

Have a pre-holiday leg waxing treatment so that you don't have to worry about taking razors and depilatory creams away with you. Nothing looks worse on the beach than hairy legs. Waxing is the most effective means of hair removal, leaving legs silky smooth. If you are a bit squeamish, do not attempt it yourself at home. Although you can buy the strips of wax, it is a difficult process and painful too if you are inexperienced in the art! However, performed by an expert at a salon, it is quick, painless and long-lasting. Afterwards, massage some special cream into your legs until signs of regrowth appear when you will need another waxing.

Moisturise your legs regularly to keep the skin smooth and supple. After bathing or showering is a good time because then your skin is warm and receptive to creams and lotions. Waxing and shaving can make it very dry and it well benefit from some pampering.

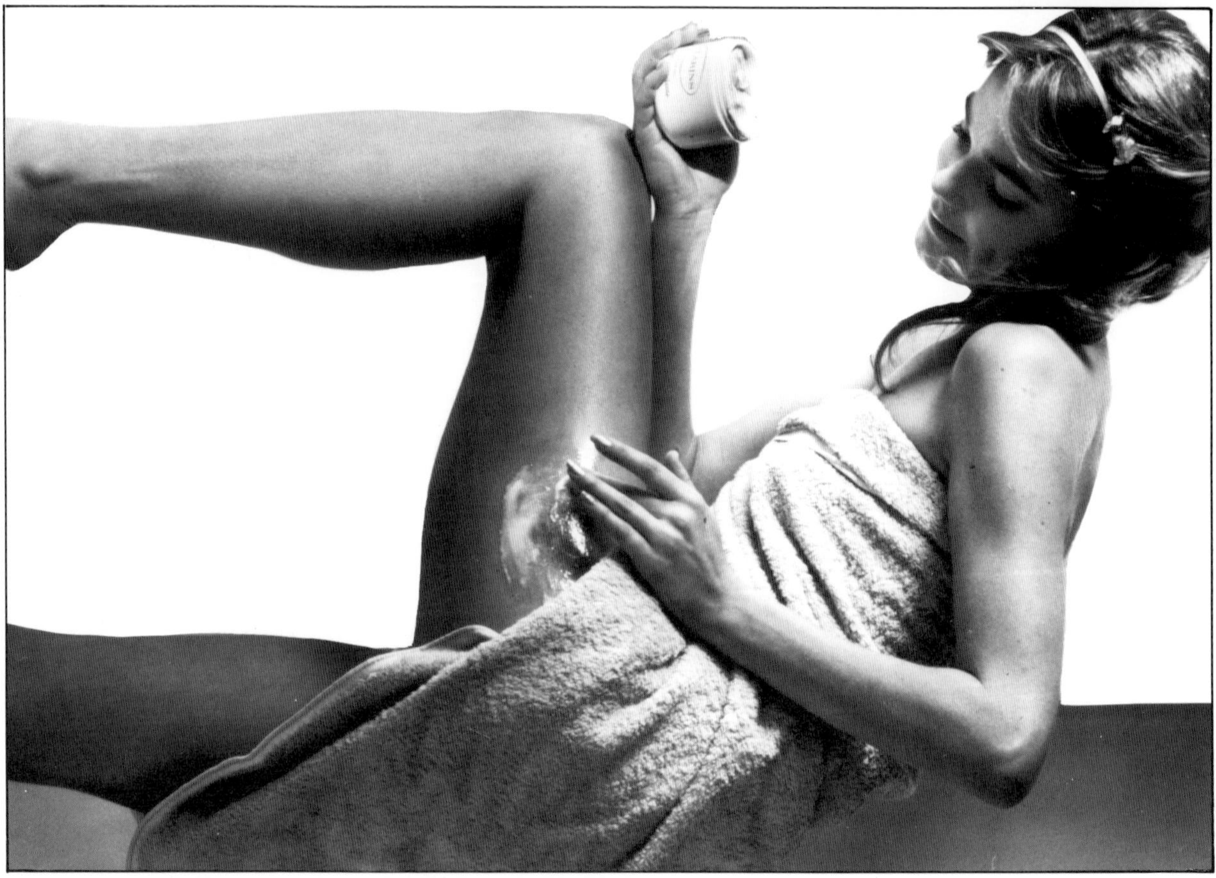

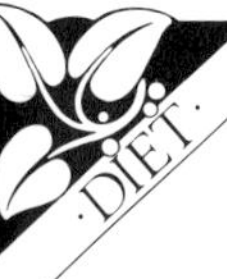

Filter your tap water for safety and purity

If you think that bottled mineral water is expensive, you can try filtering the water which comes out of your taps. It will not have the same high mineral concentration of the French quality waters, but it will be safer to drink than normal drinking water. Filtering reduces toxic iron and copper ions in the water and improves its appearance, taste and smell. It eliminates any cloudiness and gives you spring-like water at a fraction of the cost (about one-twentieth) of mineral water. Filters usually need changing after about 100 litres of tap-water so you will need some extra cartridges in reserve. Most health food stores sell water purification filters — go along and have a look today.

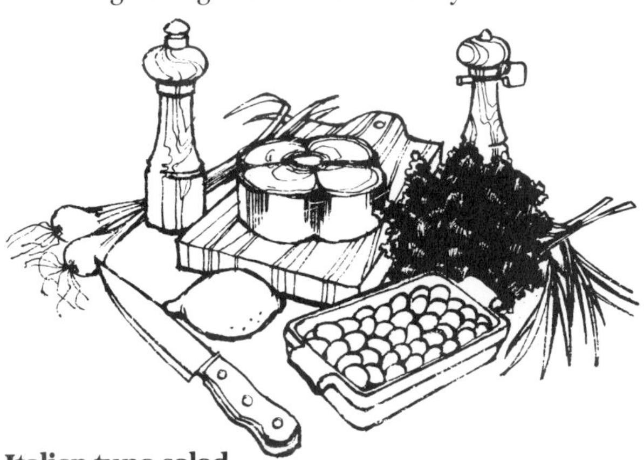

Italian tuna salad

150g/5oz cooked butter beans
75g/3oz canned tuna in brine
2 spring onions, chopped
chopped fresh chives and parsley
15ml/1 tablespoon olive oil
juice ½ lemon
salt and pepper

Mix the butter beans with tuna (drained), onion and herbs. Blend oil, lemon juice and seasoning and toss salad ingredients.

Peach and orange compôte

2 small ripe peaches
75ml/3floz unsweetened orange juice
thinly pared rind from ½ orange

Cut each peach in half and remove stones. Slice thinly and put in dish with orange juice. Cut rind into thin slivers and add to compôte. Chill. Eat with yoghurt.

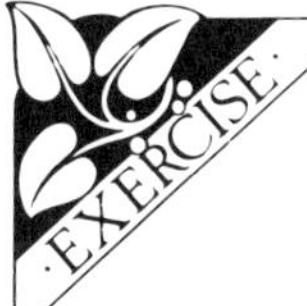

Cycle or swim your way to aerobic fitness

Choose between swimming and cycling today for your regular dose of aerobic exercise. If you enjoy your swimming, try and set yourself new hurdles every time you go to the pool. For example, add an extra length to your usual distance or swim it in a faster time. You should aim for at least 30 minutes' strenuous swimming by now — more if you feel fitter and stronger. For variety, alternate your strokes and do some pool exercises on the rail at the side to stretch out muscles and limber up. If you want to make swimming your main aerobic exercise, you might contemplate joining a club and training with other swimmers, or embarking on one of the special schemes available for adults. Ask at your local swimming baths,

Another stretching exercise for hamstring and calf muscles. Lie on back and raise legs above you. Grasp feet with hands and feel stretch in backs of legs.

Holiday tips

Treat yourself to a day at a beauty salon or health farm — most run special one day treatments for non-members and non-residents. You can usually have a massage, sauna, steam treatment, facial, manicure and exercise class for an all-inclusive special day-rate. It is well worth the money and will put the finishing touches on your beauty programme before you depart for a well-earned rest.

Why not enrol at a gym, health club, dance studio or yoga class so that you can make new friends while you exercise and learn from the professionals? Find out what facilities exist locally and you may be pleasantly surprised at how little they cost. If you find it difficult to get down to the discipline of exercising alone at home, it may be more fun to have the moral support of other like-minded people. Go along and give it a try. Even villages and small towns now have exercise, dance and aerobic classes in village halls, community centres and schools — you don't have to go to a city health club.

Day 25

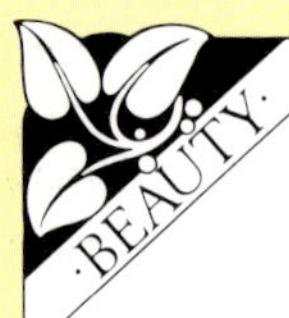

Get prepared for the hot holiday sunshine

It's high time you bought some suncare creams and lotions to take away on holiday. Before you go out shopping, decide which sun protection factor number you will need — for more information, see pages 30-31. Don't cheat and kid yourself that your skin is tougher than it really is — buy suncare products in both a higher and lower number. Then you can reap the advantages of extra protection at the beginning of your holiday, and lower the number as your tan deepens. Sunscreens not only protect you but they also allow you to tan faster. Remember also to buy a waterproof suncream for swimming, and an after-sun preparation which is soothing and moisturising at the end of a hot day.

If you have children you can purchase special protective products designed for young delicate skins. There are even sunscreens for tiny babies. Don't make false economies and imagine that all the family can share the same lotion or cream — they can't unless their skin types are all very similar and their tans are developed to exactly the same stage. Recognise that some people tan more easily than others and be guided by this when you buy suncare products.

Prepare for your holiday with a sunbed course (1). On the beach wear a good sunscreen (2) and protect your eyes with quality sunglasses (3)

3

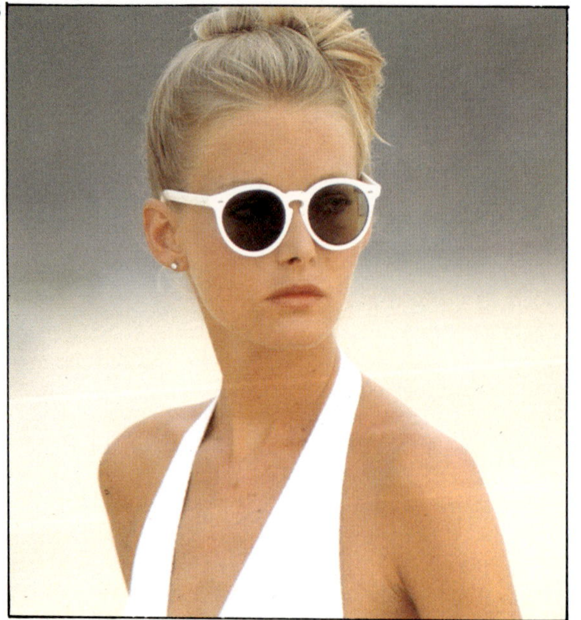

1

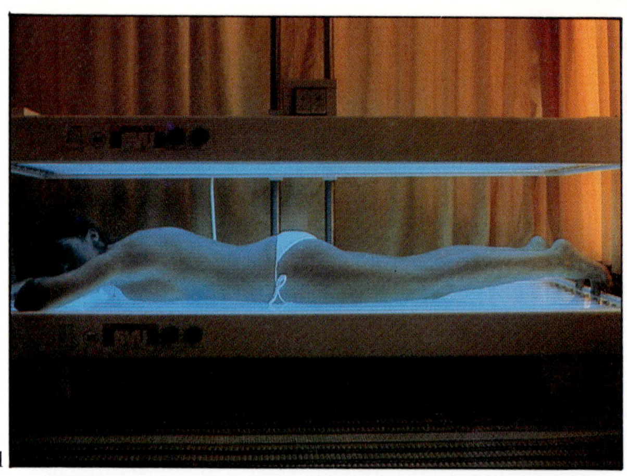

2

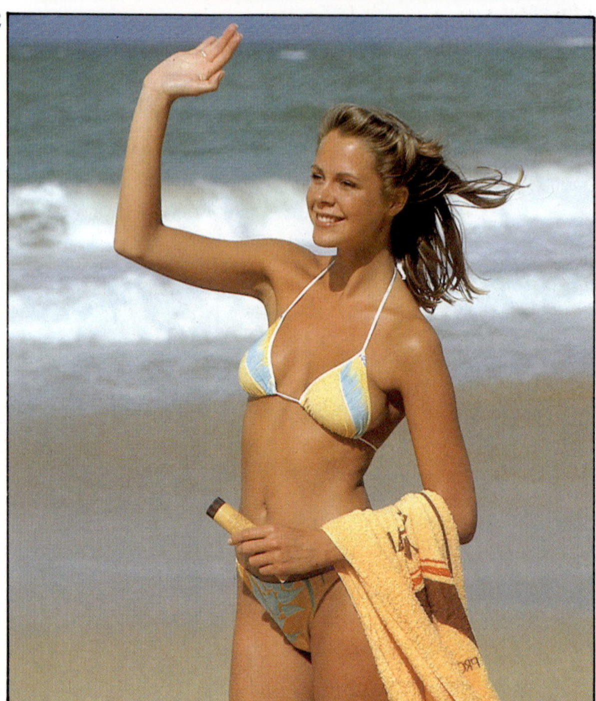

Holiday tip

Now is the time to start running down the refrigerator and your supplies of fresh food — they will not keep for the fortnight or so that you are away. Use up fresh fruit and vegetables in interesting salads, and start eating up any yoghurts, cheeses and other perishable foods. Make sure you have something put by in the freezer for a quick, easy meal when you return. You probably won't feel like cooking very much or going out shopping after a long flight or drive.

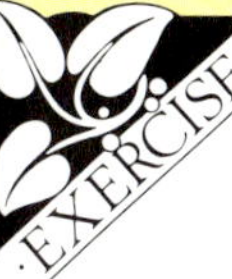

Make your muscles work for you

Another home work-out today so get warmed up and incorporate as many exercises as you can, especially the aerobic part of your programme. As you work-out, be aware of your muscles and try to control them precisely. As they get stronger and firmer you will look leaner and slimmer. This is because the exercises rhythmically lengthen and shorten your muscles, helping develop strength and flexibility. They are particularly effective for flabby areas such as the stomach or inner thighs where muscles may become flaccid due to misuse. Healthy muscles need exercise to keep them elastic — gentle stretching and rhythmic contracting will make them supple and strong. If muscles are not used they shorten, and it is only when you start to exercise and stretch them out that they ache. Of course, as you persevere and they lengthen you no longer feel any pain. After three weeks of your exercise programme, you should be feeling fitter when you perform the work-out with well-toned muscles.

Regular exercise will make you fit and supple.

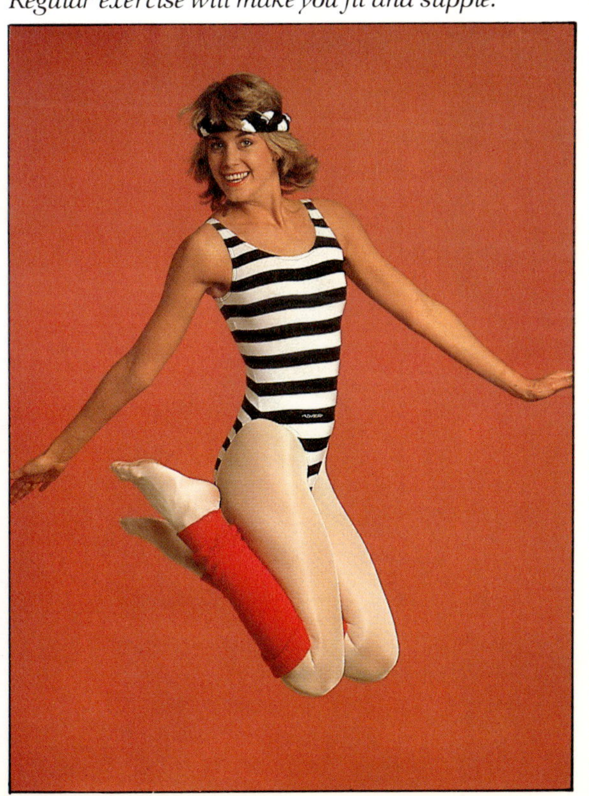

DIET

Don't suffer with a holiday tummy – take precautions

Holiday food can sometimes cause problems, especially diarrhoea, or 'Montezuma's revenge' as it is commonly known. You can get this from contaminated food or water so do take precautions with your holiday diet and be aware of potential problem foods and drinks. In some countries, especially Mexico, parts of the Mediterranean, Africa and Far East, you should sterilise drinking water by boiling it first for 10 minutes or using special sterilisation tablets. Bottled mineral waters are safe to drink, of course. Watch out for, and avoid if you are worried, ice in drinks, salads, ice-cream, milk and yoghurt — they may also be contaminated. Avoid seafood if the sea is polluted, and peel fruit and vegetables before eating or wash well in sterilised water.

If you still get an upset tummy, you will have to take an anti-diarrhoeal mixture or tablets — buy some at your local chemist and pack it in your suitcase. Mixtures of kaolin and morphine are very effective. You will also need to drink plenty of fluid to avoid dehydration. If, despite all this, the condition persists, consult a doctor without delay. You may need prescribed drugs which cannot be bought over the counter.

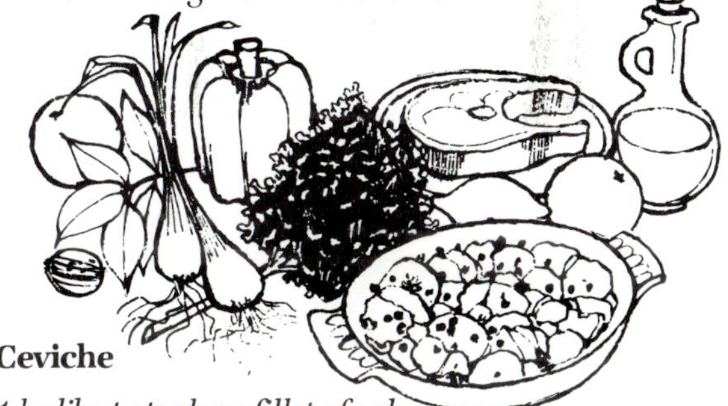

Ceviche

1 halibut steak or fillet of sole
15ml/1 tablespoon olive oil
juice of 1 lemon and 1 orange
15ml/1 tablespoon white wine vinegar
1 orange, thinly sliced
¼ green pepper, chopped
1 spring onion, chopped
bay leaf and pinch nutmeg
15ml/1 tablespoon chopped parsley

Cook the fish in oil for about 3-4 minutes each side. Remove, drain and cut into strips or chunks. Place in dish with all other ingredients except parsley. Cover and leave in refrigerator for several hours. Garnish with parsley and eat cold.

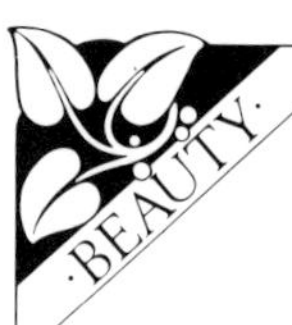

Use make-up to enhance your natural beauty

Concentrate on your face today. It's not too late to have your eyelashes dyed a darker colour if you haven't already done so — more effective and less bother than waterproof mascara. Look at your make-up and check that you really do have the right products for a holiday in the sun. Remember that softer, more subtle colours and pearly glosses and gels go well with a tan, so discard any bright blue or green powder eye shadows and brilliant orange lipsticks. Go along to a local store and ask the beautician for advice or leaf through some magazines and look at this season's colours and 'look'.

1 *After applying foundation and loose powder, concentrate on your eyes. Stroke a little powder or cream onto eyelids. Outline with liner or kohl.*
2 *Lighten the colour, fading it outwards towards brows.*

The summer effect you are trying to achieve should be healthy and natural, leaving your skin translucent and glowing. Make-up should enhance your natural beauty, making the most of your good features and playing down any weak points. It is not a mask you hide behind but a unique way of expressing your personality and making you feel more confident and attractive. Don't be afraid to change your style of make-up and to experiment with new ideas and products, especially if you have stuck with the same look for several years. What was fashionable five years ago may not suit you now, just as your pale winter make-up may look out of place on a Spanish beach in the height of summer.

Lastly, look at your make-up tools — brushes, sponges, pencil sharpeners and mirrors. Are they clean, well-washed and in good working order? You will also need some tissues for blotting make-up and lipstick.

3 *Build up layers of mascara to thicken eyelashes.*
4 *Gently apply blusher to give cheekbones definition.*
5 *Outine lips and fill in with lipstick.*
6 *The finished look is natural and pretty.*

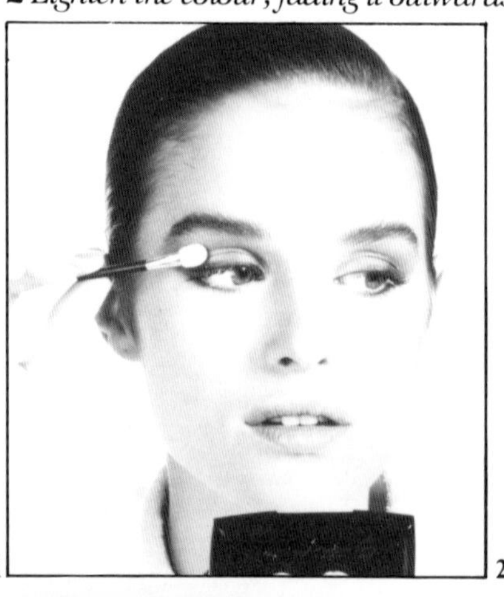
1

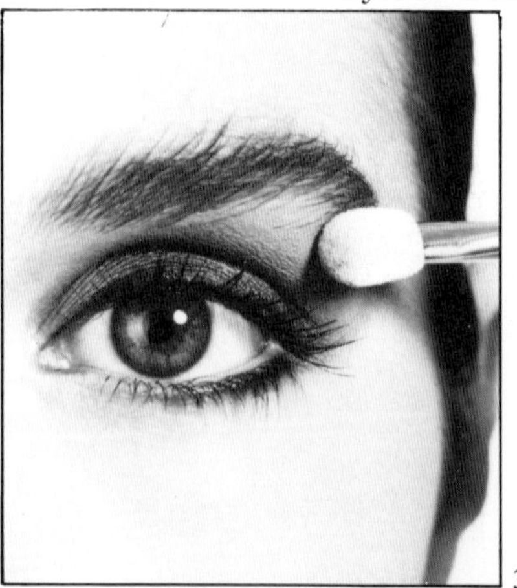
2

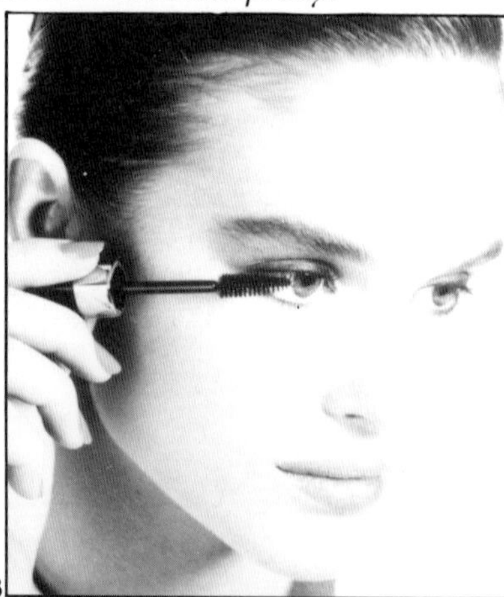
3

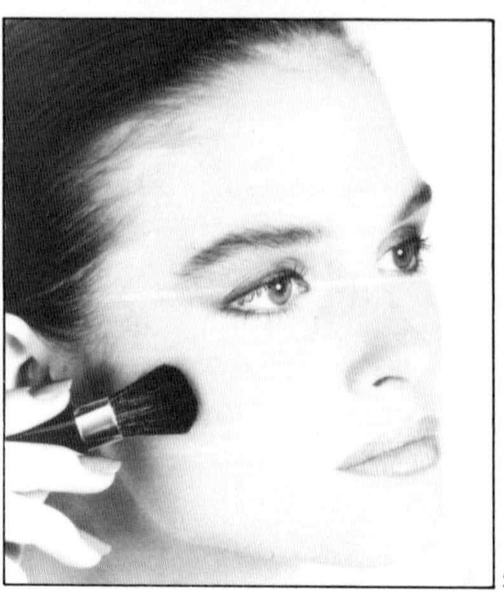
4

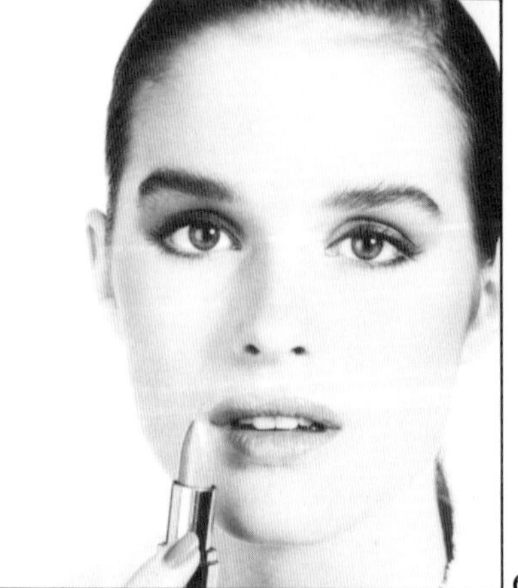
5

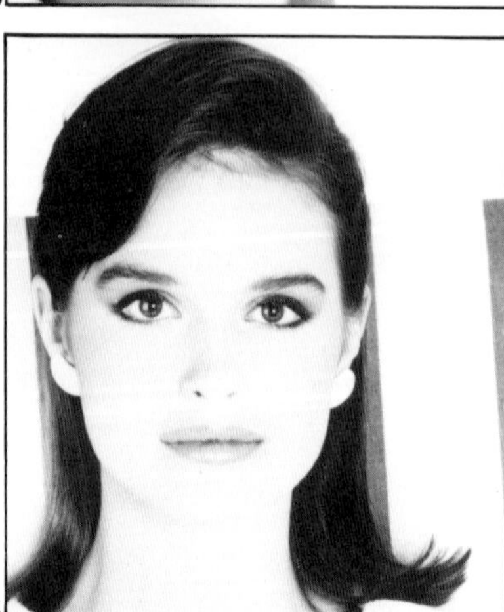
6

How to eat out the healthy way on holiday

Learn how to choose the healthy, slimming foods when you eat out in restaurants. Then you can enjoy a delicious lunch or dinner, happy in the knowledge that you have made a sensible choice. Avoid fried foods, especially French fries and deep-fried fish and vegetables in batter. Mayonnaise and rich, creamy sauces should be passed by in favour of fresh unusual salads, cold or grilled fish, shellfish and meat, pasta and rice dishes. Instead of a calorie-laden dessert or gâteau, try fresh fruit salad, fruit and cheese. With your new knowledge of nutrition, it shouldn't be difficult to pick out the most healthy items. If you are going to the Mediterranean, Latin America and the Caribbean or Asia for your holiday, you will find that the local ingredients and dishes are naturally nutritious and a lot healthier than the average Western diet. If you are self-catering, you can have fun shopping for fresh produce in colourful markets and experimenting with new foods and recipes. It might be a good idea to take a cookbook with you. There is a wide range of paperbacks to choose from — especially about Italian, Spanish, Greek and Middle Eastern food. The authors advise on how to handle and cook unfamiliar ingredients and achieve really authentic results. Then you can cook your holiday favourites when you come home afterwards, too.

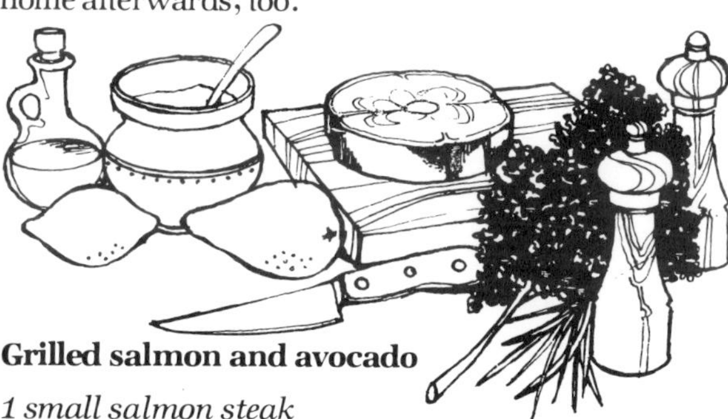

Grilled salmon and avocado

1 small salmon steak
little oil
½ small avocado pear
50ml/2floz natural yoghurt
good squeeze lemon juice
salt and pepper
few fresh chives or sprig parsley, chopped

Brush the salmon steak with oil and grill on both sides until cooked. Mash the avocado and mix with yoghurt, lemon and seasoning. Add chopped herbs and serve with salmon.

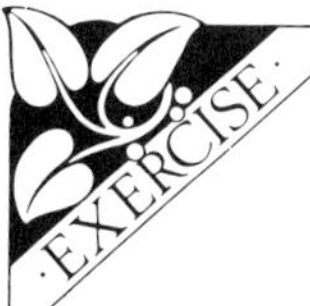

Be competitive in your running and try roller-skating

Go out jogging today — try out a different route and alternate your running pace between a gentle jog and fast strides. Really make your body work hard. If you enjoy running, it is worth keeping it up after your holiday as it is the ideal all-over conditioner and the beauty of it is that you can do it anywhere, any time. You can make your running more exciting if you decide to compete against others. Fun runs and people's marathons are becoming very popular, and even if a marathon seems too daunting for you, you might like to aim for a half-marathon or a 10K race (just over six miles). If you join an athletics club you can take part in cross-country inter-club races and track events. And if you have a real affinity for running, some special coaching may be available. Running is a great way of meeting new people and making friends.

An exciting alternative to running is roller-skating. It is hard work but most enjoyable. You will need some skates and protective shields for your knees and elbows in case you fall over. Skate to work, through the park or along special skating/cycling paths which now exist in some areas.

This aerobic exercise is an excellent way of burning up calories and although it may seem an easy option when compared with running, it is really quite strenuous if you speed-skate and negotiate hills. There are some roller skating rinks where you can go and practise before you hit the roads. Although this can be quite monotonous, it is a good way of building up speed and learning how to manoeuvre on skates. The best skates are the all-in-one boots and wheels, rather than bases with wheels attached which strap onto your normal shoes.

Holiday tip

Go shopping and buy some paperback books and magazines to read on the flight or the beach. Treat yourself to a new bikini or holiday outfit. Check your make-up bag and stock up on beauty products that are running low — you may not be able to buy your favourite mascara or cleanser on a Greek island. You will probably need new shampoo, conditioner, cotton wool balls for removing make-up, hair clips, rubber bands, soap and toothpaste. Look at the Holiday Checklist and buy what you need now.

Day 27

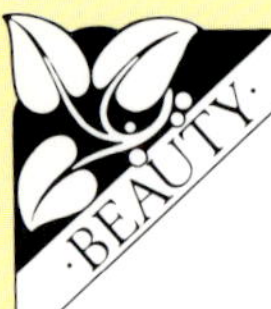

Wash and set your hair in readiness for the sun

You may not have much time to wash your hair tomorrow as you will be busy packing and making last-minute travel arrangements, so do it today instead. Shampoo and condition thoroughly, massaging your scalp really well, and then rinse until your hair is squeaky clean. To set your hair, try using a special setting lotion or mousse. Just rub it into the hair, comb through into your usual style and then blow-dry. Your hair should then look good for departure day. You can wash it again when you reach your hotel or villa, as it is bound to get sticky and dirty travelling.

If you wish to take your hair-dryer with you, check that it is lightweight and easy to pack. The best travel hairdryers are dual voltage, and you can buy a special international electrical adaptor so that you can use it in almost any country. This is available from all good electrical appliance specialist shops. You can use it for your travelling iron, too.

Don't forget to pack your hair-in-the-sun protection cream, a shower cap, bathing cap, shampoo, conditioner and some light-hold hairspray. Another useful appliance is a styling brush which dries your hair at the same time and operates off a gas cylinder.

Use a special mousse to set your hair.

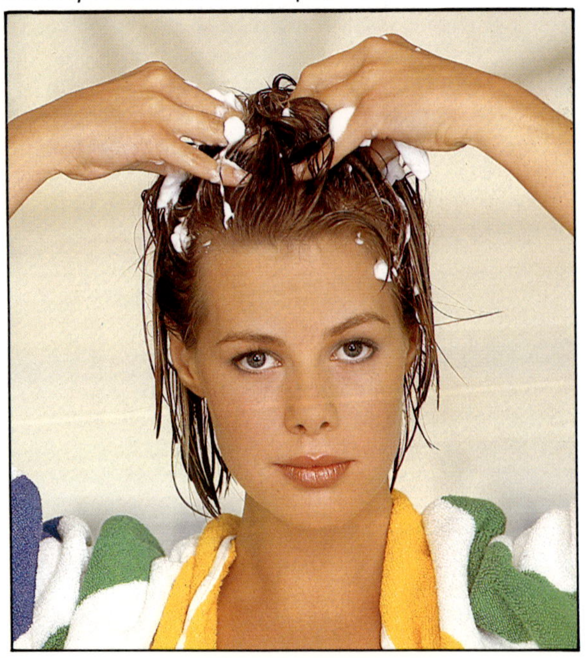

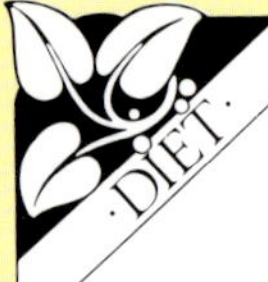

What to eat to avoid jet lag on a long flight

If you fly across several time zones, your built-in body clock may get out of alignment and you may suffer jet lag symptoms — tiredness and confusion by day, and sleeplessness at night. Sometimes it may take up to a week to adjust to your new time zone, especially if it is more than five hours time difference. If you have a long flight ahead of you, you can take positive steps to avoid jet lag and arrive at your destination feeling fresh and relaxed. The day before you depart, eat very healthy foods — salads, fresh fruit and vegetables and perhaps a little grilled white fish or chicken. Have a good night's sleep before your flight. On the plane, avoid the in-flight meals if you possibly can (not difficult!) and take some fresh fruit and a healthy snack with you in your cabin baggage. Don't drink any alcohol — stick with mineral water and fruit juices. If you can possibly do so, try and get some sleep on the plane. When you arrive at your destination at what may feel like your usual bedtime, it may still be afternoon and your hosts are raring to take you out to show you the sights and a slap-up dinner. It is best to have an early night if possible. The following day, go to bed a little later and your body clock will soon adjust and set up a new rhythm. Of course, it will have to readjust when you fly home. If you are crossing several time zones, allow at least one clear day before you go back to work or you will probably fall asleep at your desk!

Stuffed tomato platter

1 large tomato, hollowed out
50g/2oz cottage cheese
chopped chives and parsley
calabrese, chicory, spring onions and radish to garnish

To hollow out the tomato, cut off top and scoop out the seeds. Fill with cottage cheese and sprinkle with herbs. Arrange on a plate surrounded by the vegetable garnish.

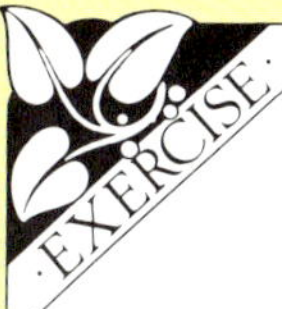

Make exercise an integral part of your lifestyle

You have a choice of swimming, cycling or working-out today.

Swimming: by now you should be well on the way to swimming 20 lengths with relative ease. If you wish to continue on a regular basis after the end of the Programme, you should aim to spend at least 20-30 minutes per session in the pool at least three times a week. Of course, if you run or work-out as well, you could limit your swimming to once or twice weekly. Always warm-up first, do the pool exercises and alternate your strokes to develop all-over fitness.

Cycling: if you have enjoyed cycling, try and make it a regular daily exercise by taking your bike, not the car or bus, to work. Otherwise, cycle four times a week for about 45 minutes per session. At weekends, you can bike out to the country for a longer, exploratory cycle — take a picnic with you in your basket or saddle-bags. Cycling is fun for all the family, and even the children can accompany you as long as you don't cycle too fast or strenuously.

Working-out: don't give up on your home work-out. Run through the exercises at least every other day to stretch out muscles and increase suppleness — they will complement your other aerobic exercises which build up endurance and stamina. To really firm up your body, try running through your usual routine but using ankle weights or dumb-bells (available from most sports shops).

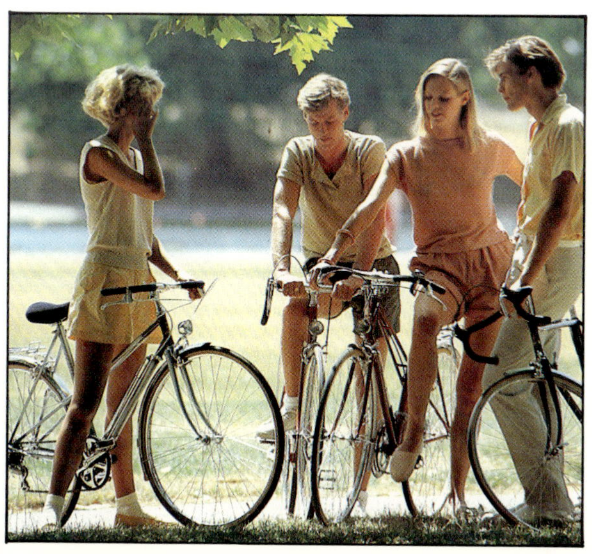

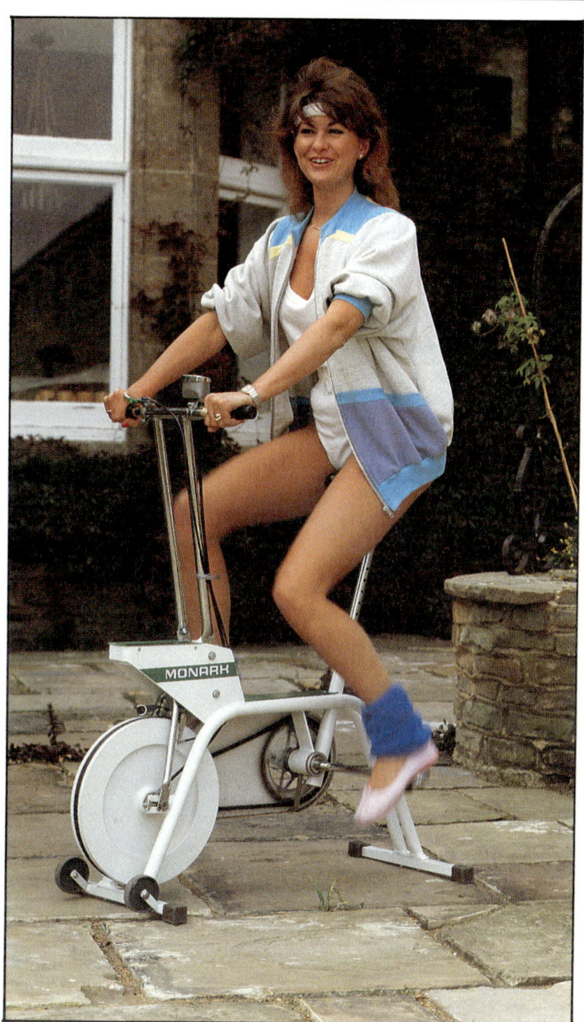

If you can't get out for a cycle, then try working-out on an exercise bike (above). You can adjust the speed to make it harder or easier depending on how energetic you feel. They are not very expensive.

Holiday tip

Visit your hairdresser for a last-minute cut and some holiday streaks and highlights. Cancel the milk and newspapers if you have not already done so. Check that all your household locks and any alarm systems are in good working order. Lock away any ladders or steps — be sure not to leave them lying around in the garden or an unlocked shed as this is just too inviting to housebreakers. Deposit any valuables in the bank. Furs can go into cold storage.

Day 28

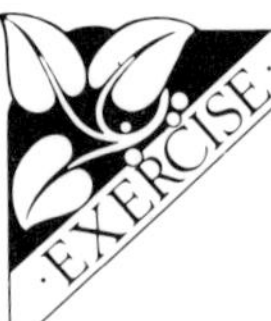

Devise your personal post-holiday fitness programme

Although it's the last day of the Programme, don't miss out on your exercise today. You won't get much tomorrow when you are busy travelling. You may not have time to go out for a swim or cycle, but try to fit in a quick run or some of your home work-out exercises. Hopefully, by now you are an addict to exercise and it has become an established part of your everyday life. To stay fit and strong you will have to exercise aerobically at least four times a week for 30 minutes per session. This will strengthen your heart and lungs and keep you slim and supple. Exercise helps you to get to know yourself and your body better, to feel more energetic and come alive. Don't stop now and throw away all the health and beauty benefits it has given you. Exercise will keep you feeling young and looking good — just continue with the sports and activities you enjoy most and set yourself new goals and obstacles to overcome. It's all very well achieving your present level of fitness, but now you have to maintain it. With all the plus factors it brings to your life — more energy and vitality, sounder sleep, a slimmer, firmer body better equipped to withstand stress, and greater powers of concentration for tackling work and personal problems — how could you possibly give up now?

On holiday, you can run, swim, cycle and choose from a wide range of watersports. When you return home, tanned and fit, devise a new exercise programme to fit into your daily routine incorporating what feels right for you and satisfies your fitness needs and natural abilities. Keep on going down the fitness road — you won't regret it.

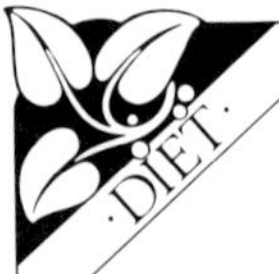

Keep on eating the right foods for a healthy lifestyle

Don't give up on your diet now, even if you have arrived at your target weight and figure. By following the general rules for healthy eating, you can maintain your new slim body and feel and look better, too. Even if you have occasional lapses when you can't resist a slice of chocolate cake or some fish and chips, as long as you eat plenty of fresh whole foods and keep your intake of processed foods to a minimum, you will be healthier. Continue eating less fats, sugar and salt; try to cook with wholemeal rather than white flour, and eat 100 per cent wholemeal bread; make sure you have high-fibre foods every day; and choose chicken and fish in preference to beef, pork and lamb. Concentrate on quick but healthy meals — you can modify and adapt your favourite recipes to the diet guidelines. For instance, substitute

Keep up your work-out classes in the coming weeks to stay fit and strong.

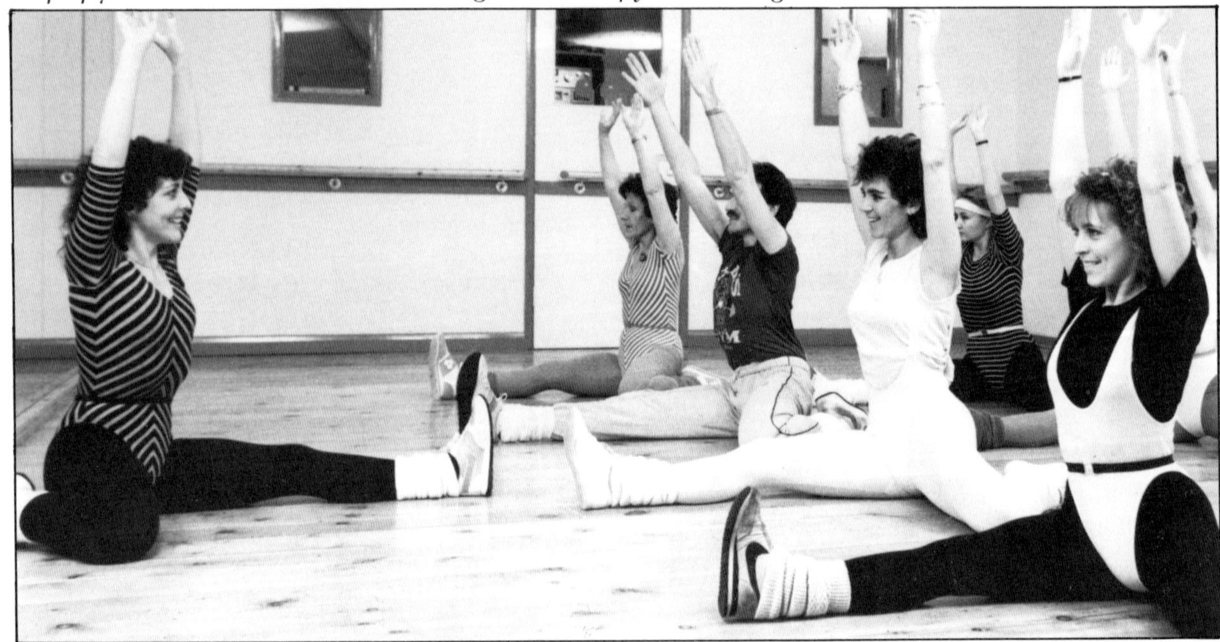

yoghurt in recipes that call for cream; make sauces with skimmed milk; make pastries and cakes with wholemeal flour; and use brown rice and wholemeal pasta in such well-known Italian dishes as risotto and spaghetti. Always read the labels on packets and cans when out shopping — put any that contain unnecessary additives firmly back on the shelf. Then you can be sure that you are buying and eating the right food for your new healthy lifestyle.

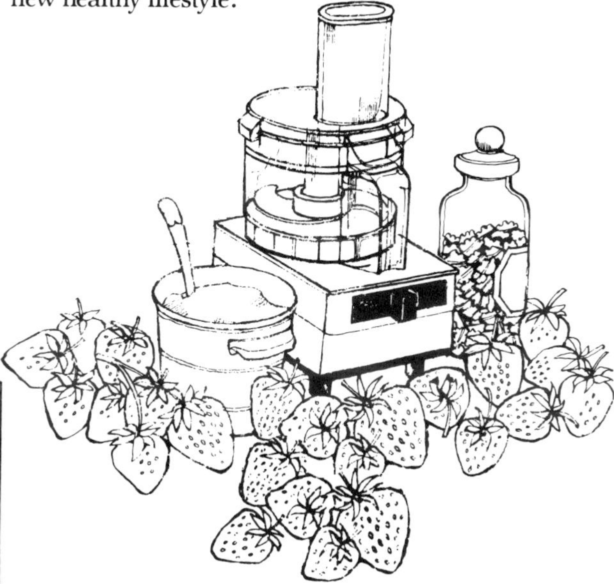

Fresh fruit fool

175g/6oz strawberries or raspberries or apricots
150ml/5floz thick natural yoghurt
10ml/2 teaspoons chopped walnuts/hazelnuts/ flaked almonds

Purée fresh strawberries or raspberries. If using apricots, cook gently over low heat until soft and juicy (add a little lemon juice if wished). Mix puréed fruit with yoghurt and chill. Decorate with chopped nuts.

Holiday tip

Pack your suitcases and bags today, using the Holiday Checklist so that you don't forget anything. Make sure that you have plenty of tissue paper for keeping creases out of clothes. When you have finished packing, lock the cases and put the keys somewhere safe in your purse or handbag. Then write out the luggage labels clearly and tie them on securely. Remember to set your alarm clock before you go to bed, or ask for an early morning phone call. It would be terrible if you overslept and missed your plane or ferry!

Make your new beauty habits last a lifetime

You have arrived at the last day of your Programme and you should be feeling and looking good. Examine your skin and weigh yourself today, and then give yourself a pat on the back for sticking to the rules. Hopefully, your efforts have been rewarded and you are fitter, slimmer with better skin and healthier hair. Don't forget to continue with your new good beauty habits when you are away on holiday and on your return, too. If you have time today in between packing, washing and ironing, last-minute shopping and travel arrangements, try to give yourself a pre-holiday face mask or exfoliating treatment. Before you go to bed, have a long soak in the bath. Add a few drops of oil to soften your skin and rub in some moisturising body lotion afterwards. Lastly, use a nourishing, rejuvenating night cream and get a good night's sleep. Before you nod off, answer these questions:

Does your skin look clearer, moister and firmer?

Does your hair look glossier and more silky?

If the answer to all these questions is "yes", then the Programme has been worthwhile and you can congratulate yourself on your dedication and self-discipline. You can look forward to your holiday in the sun, confident that you are in great shape and looking really healthy and good.

Keep your hair beautiful with regular shampooing and deep conditioning, whether it's long or short.

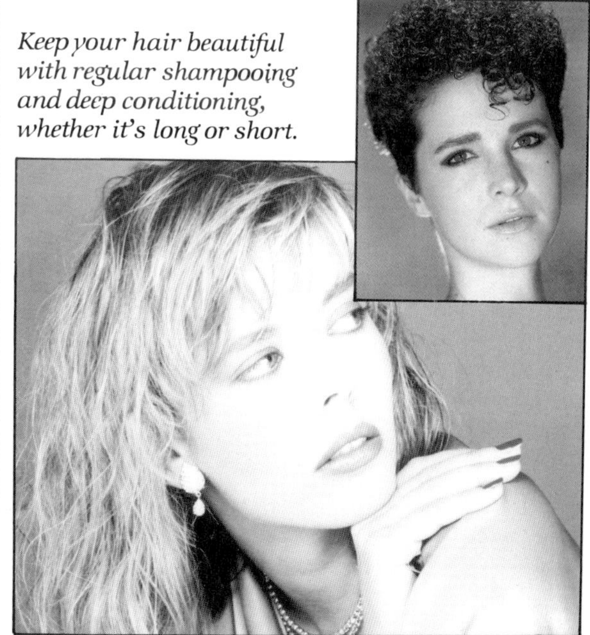

Holiday checklist

It's easy to forget things, even the basics like a toothbrush and paste, if you leave your packing to the last minute and get into a panic. If you have planned ahead and followed the tips and advice contained in the 28 Day Programme you should be superbly organised and may not need this list. However, it is a good idea to refer to it and tick off items as you pack. For more detailed advice on how to set about packing, see the special feature on pages 82-83.

Your suitcase
Double-check that you have packed the following. Use the small boxes for ticks.

1 Sponge bag
- flannel/sponge
- toothbrush and paste and floss
- skin cleanser, toner and moisturiser
- deodorant and talcum powder
- soap
- razor and tweezers
- sachet shampoos and conditioners
- hand cream
- nail scissors and manicure kit
- hair removal cream
- shower cap
- body lotion
- bath or shower foam

2 Make-up bag
- foundations and moisturisers
- concealer stick
- eye shadows/glosses, mascara, liner and pencils
- lipsticks and blushers
- packet of tissues
- cotton wool balls
- comb and brush
- nail polish and remover
- sachet face mask
- eye make-up remover
- rubber bands and hairclips

3 Sun-care
- sunscreen creams, oils or lotions
- lip salve and protective sunblock
- after-sun lotions
- sunglasses
- calamine lotion or medicated sunburn relief spray
- sunhat
- waterproof sunscreen

4 First-aid
- waterproof plasters in assorted sizes
- pain-relief tablets
- antiseptic cream
- anti-diarrhoea tablets/medicine
- antacid or indigestion tablets
- anti-malarial tablets
- throat lozenges
- water sterilisation tablets
- tampons
- petroleum jelly

5 Electrical goods
- dual-voltage hair dryer with adapter/plug
- heated rollers
- travel-iron
- travelling alarm clock
- heated curling tongs
- ladyshave

6 Clothes
- bras, pants, tights and slips
- lightweight cotton nightdress/pyjamas
- cotton robe/dressing gown
- sundresses/day dresses
- evening dresses
- short and long skirts
- cool tops/T-shirts/blouses
- bikinis and swimsuits
- beach robe
- lightweight jacket
- fold-away lightweight mac
- warm cardigan/shawl/pullover
- jeans/evening trousers
- shorts
- espadrilles/sandals/flip-flops
- evening shoes

7 Sportsgear
- running shoes/trainers
- tennis shoes
- leotard
- tracksuit
- running shorts and T-shirts
- tennis whites
- tennis racket
- snorkel and flippers
- socks
- swimming cap

continued on page 80

In case you forget to remember

Remember to...

Before you go away, remember to do the following things in order to put your mind at ease while you're on holiday and make sure that your home is properly looked after in your absence.

1 Tell the neighbours that you are going away and for how long. Give them a telephone number or an address at which you can be contacted in case of emergencies.

2 Ask them to go in and water any houseplants, mow the lawn, water the garden, turn lights on to deter housebreakers. Deposit a key with them before you leave in case of emergencies.

3 Cancel the milk. You don't want bottles and cartons piling up on your doorstep — a sure sign to criminals that you are away.

4 Arrange for mail to be readdressed if wished. Ask the post office for details.

5 Cancel any newspapers that are normally delivered.

6 Lock all doors and make sure that windows are properly secured.

7 Move all houseplants away from windowsills — they may wilt in bright sunlight. If possible, buy an automatic watering system for them.

8 Turn off the water and gas. Pull out all electrical plugs, leaving only the freezer switched on.

9 Make sure that there is no fresh food in the cupboards or fridge that can go mouldy in your absence — throw it away.

10 Ask the police to keep an eye on the house.

11 Give the garden a really thorough watering.

12 Take any pets to the kennels/cattery or friends to be looked after.

13 Deposit any jewellery or valuables in the bank for safe keeping.

14 Lock up the garage and any outside sheds and buildings.

15 Pay any outstanding household bills. You don't want to return home to find that the phone or electricity have been cut off. There is always a reconnection charge.

16 Collect any clothes from the cleaners.

17 Cancel any deliveries of oil or coal which are due to arrive while you are away. Fix a new delivery date for when you return.

18 Plan and get ready any food for your journey.

19 Arrange an early-morning alarm call.

20 Turn on the alarm system if you have one.

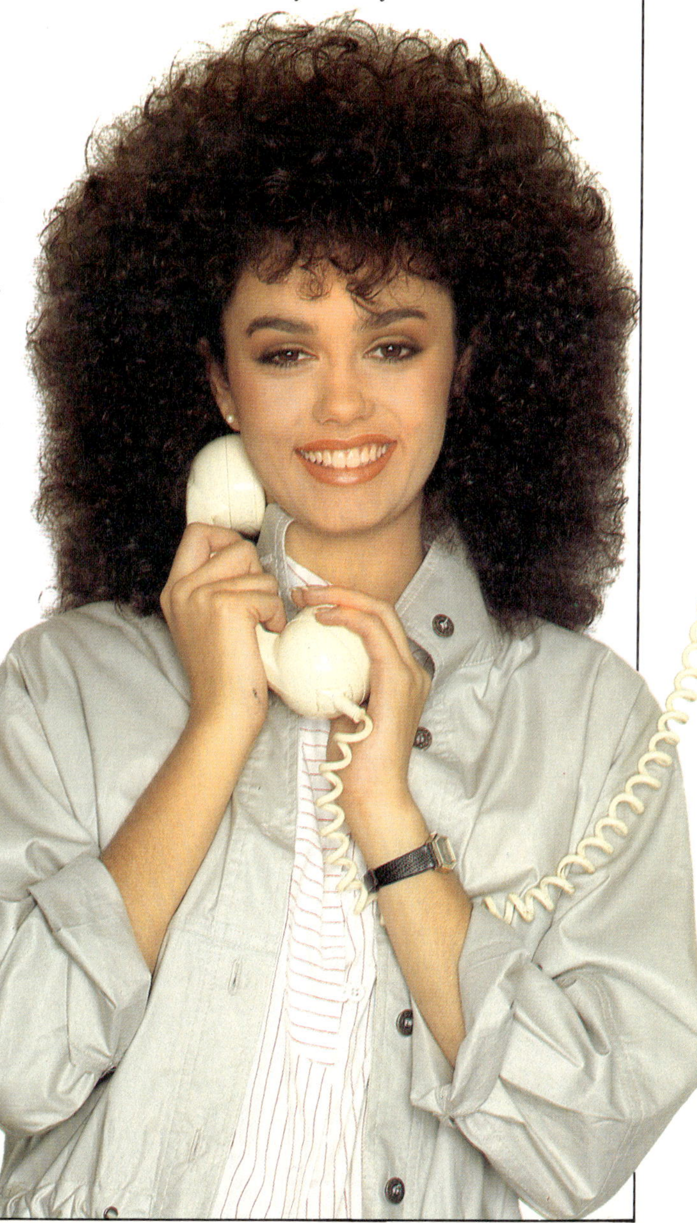

Holiday checklist

8 Accessories

- long scarves ☐
- belts ☐
- costume jewellery to match outfits ☐
- hair slides and combs ☐
- foldaway umbrella ☐
- evening bag ☐

9 Extras

- washing powder (small packet) ☐
- sewing repair kit ☐
- penknife ☐
- insect repellant ☐
- contraceptive pills ☐
- corkscrew/can opener ☐
- phrase book/dictionary ☐
- mini clothes line ☐
- beach towel ☐
- inflatable lilo ☐
- beachbag and mat ☐
- guidebooks ☐
- hair rollers ☐

Your handbag and cabin baggage

Check that you have packed the following for the journey:

- tissues ☐
- eau-de-cologne/soothing wet-wipes ☐
- books/magazines ☐
- camera and films ☐
- stereo headset radio/cassette player ☐
- notepad and pens ☐
- cosmetics and hand mirror ☐
- hairbrush/comb ☐
- spare contact lenses/spectacles ☐
- address book and diary ☐
- jewellery ☐
- wallet/purse and money ☐
- travellers cheques ☐
- passport ☐
- ticket document wallet ☐
- credit cards ☐
- international driving licence ☐
- thermos flask of drink ☐
- plastic bottled mineral water ☐
- fresh fruit and healthy snack ☐
- safety pins ☐
- boiled sweets to stop ears popping ☐
- travel sickness pills ☐
- any medication ☐
- insurance forms/premiums ☐

Everybody wants an annual holiday but the choice is so overwhelming nowadays that you might have difficulty deciding on where you want to go and in what sort of accommodation you wish to stay. Obviously your final decision will be guided by how much money you can afford to spend and what sort of person you are — sporty, fun-loving, sunworshipper, exercise fanatic, adventurous or lazy. Do you like roughing-it under canvas or a starlit sky, or do you prefer to stay in a luxury hotel? Here's a brief guide to the different holiday choices on offer, which you can either plan and organise yourself, or book through a tour operator as a complete package. Ask your travel agent.

1 Staying in a hotel

If you want to be waited on and looked after for a couple of weeks, then this kind of holiday is best as no self-catering, cleaning or any of the other usual chores are involved — everything is done for you. You can either make a booking at the hotel of your choice and arrange the air travel or motor there yourself, or you can book a package deal. Every year the major tour operators and smaller more specialised companies, too, produce colour brochures of their whole range of summer holidays complete with pictures of the resorts, individual hotels and prices. Most hotels offer a full- or half-board deal, depending on whether you wish to eat your meals there or eat one meal a day out at a restaurant or enjoy a picnic on the beach. Hotels are usually graded by tour operators according to their location and amenities. For instance, an expensive first-class hotel will probably have an international restaurant, swimming pool, tennis courts, hairdresser, beauty salon, shopping arcade, and maybe even its own private beach. Smaller, more inexpensive hotels and pensions will have less extensive amenities. Bedrooms vary, too, and you will have to pay more for a sea view, own bathroom and cocktail bar, for example.

2 Apartments, villas and cottages

Self-catering holidays are very popular, especially among families with young children. If you don't mind doing all the work on holiday, they usually work out much cheaper than staying in a hotel but you have to allow for the additional costs of buying food. Sometimes a cleaning or maid service is provided but you may have to pay more for this unless it is included in the quoted price. If you prefer more space and freedom to move about and make a noise, then this type of holiday may offer a better deal than staying in a hotel. There are companies which specialise in this type of holiday, and most big tour operators also offer villa and apartment holidays with the airfare thrown in. If you want to really get away from it all, you might consider renting a remote farmhouse or cottage in the wilds of Tuscany or Provence, for example. Ask your travel agent for a range of brochures which cover your preferred destinations. Self-catering holidays can be great fun if you enjoy buying and cooking food from the local market and trying out new recipe ideas. And if you don't fancy cooking, you can always try the regional dishes in a neaby restaurant. It is more difficult to eat out with the locals if you buy an all-in full-board arrangement in a big hotel which may serve the sort of food you are used to eating at home, anyway.

This type of holiday is well-suited to children who may be faddy about eating hotel food or have embarrassing table manners when very young. It is a strain keeping them on their best behaviour all the time and it is easier to live your normal family life in a rented villa or apartment. Some complexes provide special babysitting and listening services so that you can go out and enjoy yourself in the evenings without worrying about the kids.

3 Caravanning
Some people enjoy hitting the open road and pulling their little home for two weeks behind them, moving from site to site rather than staying in one place. Others like to fly, drive or take the train and hire a caravan on a special site. Either you're an addict or you see caravanning as an economical way to take a holiday. Sites vary enormously in the facilities on offer — some are quite primitive whereas others have shops, a supermarket, night-club, laundry, swimming pool, restaurants, TV rooms, first-class showers and bathrooms, mains-water connections and gas and electricity piped to your caravan. You may wish to pay more for all these modern comforts or you may prefer a cheaper, less developed site.

4 Camping
If your idea of heaven on earth is a tent pitched in a lush green meadow beside a small stream or a modern campsite overlooking the beach, then a camping holiday is a cheap option. You don't have to buy an expensive tent and all the equipment unless you are really under the spell. You can either rent one from a camping specialist hire shop or even hire a tent on a site. Tents range from fairly primitive collapsible affairs to the tubular frame luxury variety complete with awnings, sewn-in groundsheets and roof insulation. A good-quality new tent should last for years, but you can also pick up some worthwhile second-hand bargains from people who lost the bug or are planning to buy an even bigger and better tent.

If something goes wrong....
What do you do if your journey does not go as smoothly as planned? Here's some advice on how to deal with the sort of mishaps and problems you may encounter.

1 The flight's delayed
Unfortunately, this happens all too often, especially in bad weather conditions or when there is industrial action by airport or airline employees. If you suspect that there may be a delay, phone the airport before you leave and find out if your flight is affected and how late it may be. However, it is still a good idea to turn up and check-in just in case the situation improves and the plane leaves on time after all. But you can take along some extra magazines or food to pass the time while you wait. Be as patient as you possibly can and listen out for bulletins. Some major airlines will pay for a meal or even book you into a hotel overnight if there is going to be a long wait, but this is highly unlikely if you are flying out on a package or charter. Although you can't insure against bad weather, it is possible to take out a policy against delay through industrial action.

2 The flight is overbooked
Although you may be able to resign yourself to a delay, it is hard to stay cool if you arrive to check-in for a seat that is already paid for and you are told that the plane is overbooked and you will be allocated another seat on the next available flight. Basically, you can't ever be sure that your booking is safe — it is normal policy to overbook in order to fill seats as lots of people don't turn up for their flight. You can usually avoid this happening to you by checking-in early, but if you are unlucky you can insist that the airline gives you complimentary meals and accommodation if necessary while waiting for the next available seat.

3 Your luggage is lost
Don't panic if your baggage is lost in transit and never appears on the carousel. It might have been overlooked in the hold, be waiting for boarding back at home, or been misrouted to the wrong destination. Tell the airline immediately and they will try to trace it for you. It nearly always turns up. Go to the lost-luggage desk and give them all the details. Insist that they send it to your hotel or wherever you're staying when it eventually arrives. To guard against any inconvenience caused, take some washing things and a change of clothing in your cabin baggage. At least you'll be able to feel clean and fresh after arriving at the hotel.

Travelling light

Well-seasoned travellers always travel light, packing only the bare essentials and *never* cluttering up their luggage with unnecessary things. It is a good idea to plan your packing in advance in order to avoid last-minute panics. So about a week before your departure date, sit down and work out a list. There are several things you need to consider:

1 What will the climate be like — warm or very hot?
2 What sort of nightlife will there be?
3 Which sports and activities will be on offer?

Your answers will help determine your choice of clothes, accessories and sportsgear. For more advice on what to pack and a handy list to tick off as you go along, consult the Holiday Checklist.

Have a look at the clothes you plan to take and check them for stains, missing buttons, broken zip fasteners and falling hems. All these things can be rectified.

Get carried away by luggage

Lightweight luggage, especially collapsible reinforced bags, is best for flying. Lighter and more colourful than conventional suitcases, these bags are strong and durable, often made of nylon or tough woven canvas and reinforced at the points of strain. Many have shoulder straps to keep your hands free and are even small enough to qualify as cabin baggage on aircraft.

If you prefer suitcases, then choose ones which are strong and sturdy in leather-look vinyl or canvas with padded handles for comfortable carrying. Expensive luggage looks classy when new but it is likely to get knocked about by airport baggage handlers.

Although most international airports provide free trolleys, it's a good idea to invest in a pair of attachable wheels which can be strapped on to your suitcase and take the weight off your arms.

Always lock your suitcase so that it can't spring open as it comes off the carousel or be tampered with in transit. Tie some labels to the handle and attach some stickers with your name, destination and home address printed clearly on them. This is essential in the case of loss or the eventuality of it being loaded onto the wrong plane. Then if it does turn up in Malaga instead of Athens, there is a good chance that it will be returned safely to you. Remove any old labels and check that zips are in good working order.

Another good tip is to add your own personal touch of identification by tying some brightly coloured braid or ribbon to the handles. This will avoid potential mix-ups on airport carousels.

Baggage allowances

Check with your ticket and travel documents to find out your free baggage allowance for the flight. Allowances vary on international and European routes with some Transatlantic carriers permitting two pieces of luggage only of any weight. If there is a weight allowance, weigh your cases carefully so that you are not liable for an expensive excess baggage charge. In addition to your free allowance, you can also take free of charge as cabin baggage, a handbag, umbrella, camera, duty-free goods, reading matter, a carry-cot and babyfood.

Send'em packing

Always pack bulky things first — shoes, hairdryer, travel-iron, sponge bag — either at the bottom of a soft bag or along the hinged sides of a sturdy suitcase. Fill the gaps in between with soft things like underwear, tights, socks, scarves, belts and handkerchiefs. On top, arrange skirts, trousers and jackets, all carefully colour-coordinated, and lastly dresses and shirts.

To minimise creasing, fold all your clothes carefully in large sheets of crisp tissue paper with plenty of paper between folds. Drip-dry, permanent-press clothes are perfect for holiday packing as they crease less and wash easily in the absence of an iron. However, if your clothes still get creased despite taking precautions, you can always try hanging them up above a hot steamy bath to help any creases drop out, or buy a small travel-iron.

Even if you're going to a hot climate, pack at least one warm jacket or pullover as tropical evenings can be cool and some days colder than you anticipate. Also, take extra plastic carrier bags for dirty laundry, packing shoes and holiday shopping expeditions. Make sure that shampoos, make-up, suncare lotions and washing things are all in leakproof, unbreakable plastic bottles to avoid spillage. Pack them into a zipped-up sponge bag. Never pack inflammable lighter fluid or aerosols which can leak at high altitudes in your suitcase. Finally, cover everything with a large sheet of polythene before closing the bag/case just in case any rain water leaks in through a faulty catch or zip.

Bon voyage!

Wear loose, comfortable, crease-resistant clothes for travelling so that you arrive at your holiday destination fresh, neat and cool. Store your in-flight needs in a handy shoulderbag. You will need a book or magazine to pass the time, some refreshing wet-wipes, a snack of fruit and a plastic bottle of mineral water to beat jet-lag on a long flight, plus any jewellery or valuables which should never be packed in your stow-away luggage as they cannot be covered by insurance if lost or damaged in transit. Wear soft, comfortable shoes as feet tend to swell at high altitudes.

Smart suitcases (opposite top) always look impressive when travelling, but you may find lightweight bags in strong colourful fabrics (bottom) best for cabin baggage.

Get precision packed

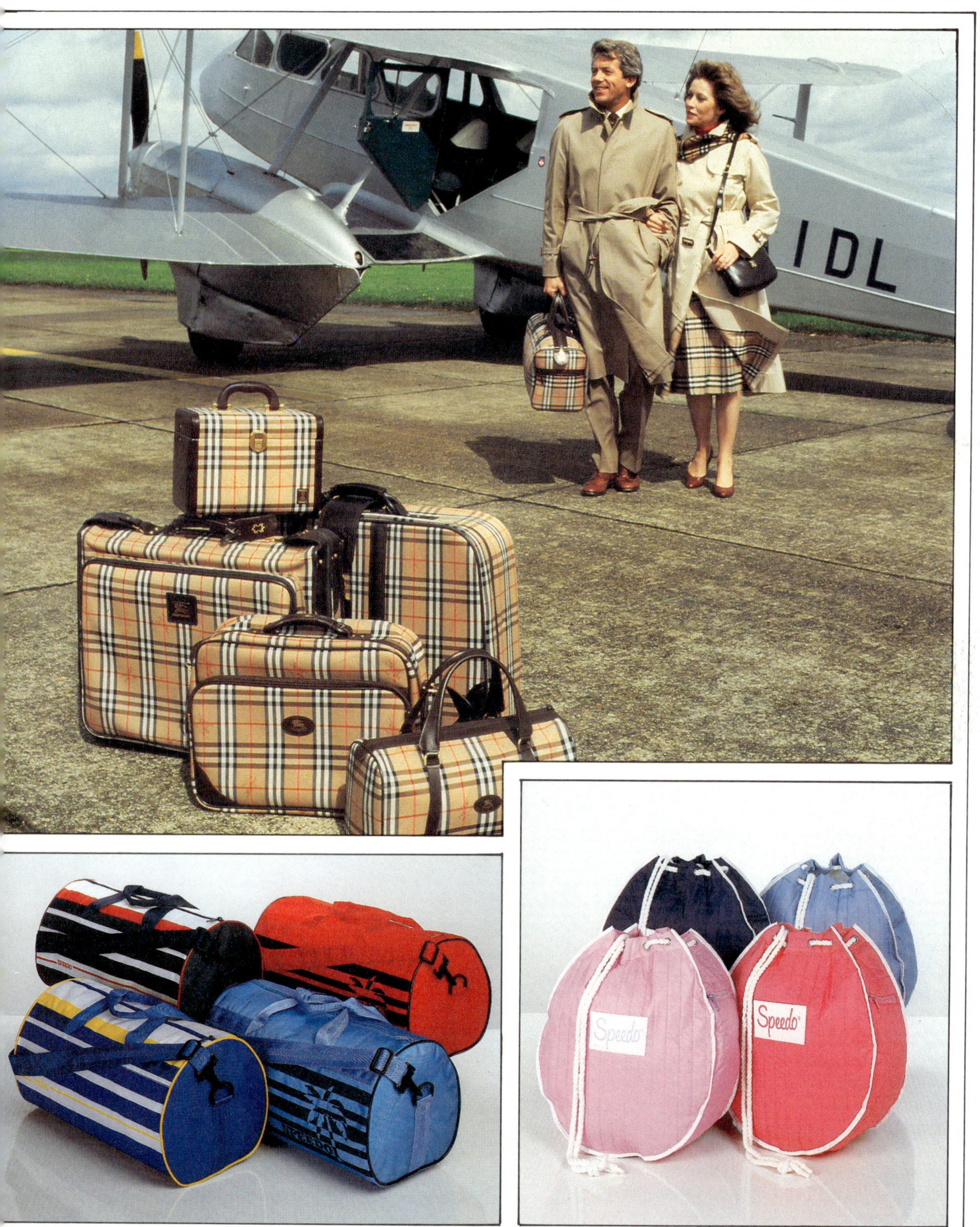

Holiday reference guide

By the time you reach the end of the Programme you should be fit and healthy for your trip but there may be other health factors that you should take into account such as medical insurance in case of accident or illness, vaccinations and some basic precautions to avoid ill health on holiday.

Vaccination

Immunisation to protect you against virulent diseases is compulsory for entering some countries and advisable for others — check with your travel agent. Your doctor can vaccinate you against tetanus, typhoid, poliomyelitis, infectious hepatitis and cholera. Yellow fever vaccinations are usually given only at special centres. However, you will only need this vaccination if you are travelling to Panama, South America and central and tropical Africa. It is contracted from an infected mosquito's bite. Here's a short list of diseases and the areas in which they may be caught:

1 Cholera is usually caused by contaminated water, and the main risk areas are Africa, the Middle East, Asia and the Far East. Even if you are travelling to North African resorts — in Morocco and Egypt, for instance, or to Turkey — it is recommended that you should have a cholera jab at least 10 days before you depart. If you are having another live vaccine such as polio, you should leave a gap of at least three weeks between immunisations.
2 Malaria may result from an infected *anopheles* mosquito's bite. If you are visiting North Africa, the Middle East, Central and South America or Asia, you should take a course of anti-malarial tablets before, during and even after your holiday. Check with your doctor a week before leaving.
3 Poliomyelitis is still around in southern Europe as well as the Middle East, Africa, Asia, the Far East, Central and South America. Even if you were vaccinated as a child, it is a good idea to have a top-up dose just to be on the safe side. It is quite painless nowadays as it is given orally on a lump of sugar. Even if you are travelling to Spain, Gibraltar, Malta, Cyprus, Madeira, Turkey or the Carribbean islands, it makes sense to have a polio booster.
4 Typhoid immunisation is advisable for anywhere other than northern Europe and North America, New Zealand and Australia. You can catch typhoid from contaminated food or water, and vaccination is essential for newly developed Mediterranean resort areas and camping/caravan sites. You will need two injections, preferably separated by an interval of four weeks. So go to your doctor about six weeks before your departure date. If you got a last-minute holiday booking, you can make do with only 10 days between jabs, but this covers you for one year instead of three.
5 Yellow fever is a disease confined to the tropics. Immunisation is compulsory for Central Africa and is recommended in South America, too. You should be vaccinated at least 10 days before your departure date and this will give you 10 years' cover.
For more information on vaccinations, contact your travel agent or government health department.

Medical insurance

You can take this out against personal accident or medical treatment while you are abroad on holiday. Most insurance companies have special inexpensive holiday policies, which usually cover medical and emergency expenses up to £100,000 (about 130,000 US dollars). You should make sure that an air ambulance for repatriation (flying you home after an accident or illness) is included in the policy.

For North America, you may need a different policy — your insurance broker or travel agent will advise you. Read the small print carefully when taking out any policy, especially any exclusions for which the insurer will not pay — you may find that the policy has less scope than you thought. For example, it may not cover a diving or mountaineering accident. You may have to take out a separate policy for Personal Accident.

Reciprocal health arrangements exist between EEC (European Economic Community) countries and you will need to fill in the necessary application forms before you go away (available from local health offices). However, you may be entitled only to reduced, free, medical treatment so check up on what you are getting and if necessary take out additional private medical insurance.

Basic health precautions

You can avoid illness and health problems by taking the following precautions:
1 Take care in the sun — use sunscreens and blocks to prevent burning (see pages 30-31) If you want to enjoy your holiday and get a beautiful golden tan, you must take your sunbathing gradually and carefully.
2 Be sensible in excessive heat — do not spend long periods outside in extreme heat if you are unused to high temperatures and humidity. Nor should you exercise strenuously at the hottest times of the day. Protect your head with a sunhat in hot sunshine. Heat exhaustion is a real danger if you lose a lot of fluid through sweating and do not replace it with sufficient non-alcoholic drinks. If you feel dizzy, nauseous, cold and clammy, then lie down and rest in a cool place. Drink plenty of water to replace lost fluids. If you do not take care, exhaustion sometimes gives way to heat stroke which may require medical attention.

3 Drink plenty of fluids in hot climates — these will stop your body becoming dehydrated. Limit your alcohol intake, though, as this may dehydrate you further. Mineral water and fruit juices are cooling and refreshing in warm weather.
4 Beware of contaminated food and water — in countries where standards of hygiene and sanitation are poor, especially Africa, Central and South America, Asia and even parts of the Mediterranean, you should take a few precautions. Drink only boiled or sterilised water, don't have iced drinks, and avoid milk, yoghurt, and ice-cream if you fear that the water may be suspect. Peel all fruit and vegetables.

Bites and stings

You may be unlucky enough to encounter one of several unfamiliar animals, insects and sea-creatures while you're on holiday. Although your chances of doing so are very low indeed, it is a good idea to know what to do if the situation arises:
Sea urchins: if you step on one of these on the rocks or beach, its long black spines may become embedded in your feet. Treat with magnesium sulphate paste. Better still, look where you're treading and wear shoes.
Jellyfish: these are often found in warm waters so be on the look-out when paddling or swimming. They look like transparent plates of jelly with waving strands. If stung, apply some cooling calamine lotion to the affected area, or ice packs and cold compresses. Fever may develop in extreme cases — if so, seek medical advice without delay.
Rabies: this horrible disease still occurs in Europe and other parts of the world, so don't pat strange dogs or fondle stray cats. If you are scratched or bitten by any dog or cat, try to exchange names and addresses with the owner to be on the safe side. Then if the animal contracts the disease within a fortnight he can let you know immediately and you can be vaccinated. If you suspect that an animal is rabid, report to the nearest hospital straight away for treatment. Even a normal bite should be washed thoroughly and a tetanus injection given. Don't think it couldn't possibly happen to you and neglect to follow these precautions — rabies is a killer and it is rare for anyone to recover from it.

Hangover

This is a common holiday disorder, especially among lovers of good food, wine and late nights out dancing. If you regret all your self-indulgence in the morning, you can try one of several things — while some people swear by a glass of fresh orange juice, others prefer to take a foul concoction of Fernet Branca or a fizzy antacid mixture. The headache will soon go if you take a couple of painkillers. But it is better to avoid a hangover in the first place by drinking less and only with food, watering down your wine with mineral water or having a large glass of milk before you set out for a night on the town. Vodka and gin are preferable to whisky, brandy and port when it comes to preventing hangovers; and drinking large quantities of water before going to bed may stop dehydration and that awful 'morning after the night before' feeling the following day.

Eyes, ears, throat and teeth

Swimming can sometimes irritate eyes and ears and lead to throat infections, too. Wear goggles if so and a tight-fitting swimming cap. Eye drops or soothing cotton wool pads soaked in cold tea or witch hazel will revive tired, inflamed eyes. Antiseptic eardrops help prevent ear infections if you develop a slight discharge. Gargling regularly with saltwater is beneficial to toothache and throat infections. Take some toothache tincture with you just in case — oil of cloves is very effective — and some throat lozenges, too.

If you're pregnant

It's perfectly safe to go away on holiday while you're pregnant, but most airlines require a letter from your doctor stating that you are well enough to travel if you are more than 28 weeks. Of course, if you had a miscarriage in an earlier pregnancy, you have high blood pressure or some other pregnancy-related medical problem, it is better to stay at home and wait for a holiday after your baby is born. Flying in late pregnancy is tiring and stressful, and has even been known to bring on premature labour. Obviously it is better and safer for you to have your baby in a modern well-equipped hospital than 30,000 feet up in the sky in cramped conditions with inexperienced help. If you are travelling in the early months of pregnancy, make sure that you wear loose, comfortable clothes and take some slippers to allow for swollen feet. Pack your card in case there are health problems and you need to consult a doctor. It will record all relevant details concerning your pregnancy. If you are on a plane or boat, get up regularly and go for a walk to increase circulation in your legs and pelvic area. If you are immobile in a car or coach, practise rolling your feet in circles and writing imaginary words in the air with them.

Before you depart, ask your doctor which injections it is safe for you to have and which travel sickness pills are best. Obviously, it is better for your health and the baby's sake if you do not take any drugs at all and avoid vaccination, too, as it may increase the risk of miscarriage in the first three months. Although cholera and typhoid vaccination are relatively safe you should not visit countries for which yellow fever immunisation is essential.

Keep fit on holiday

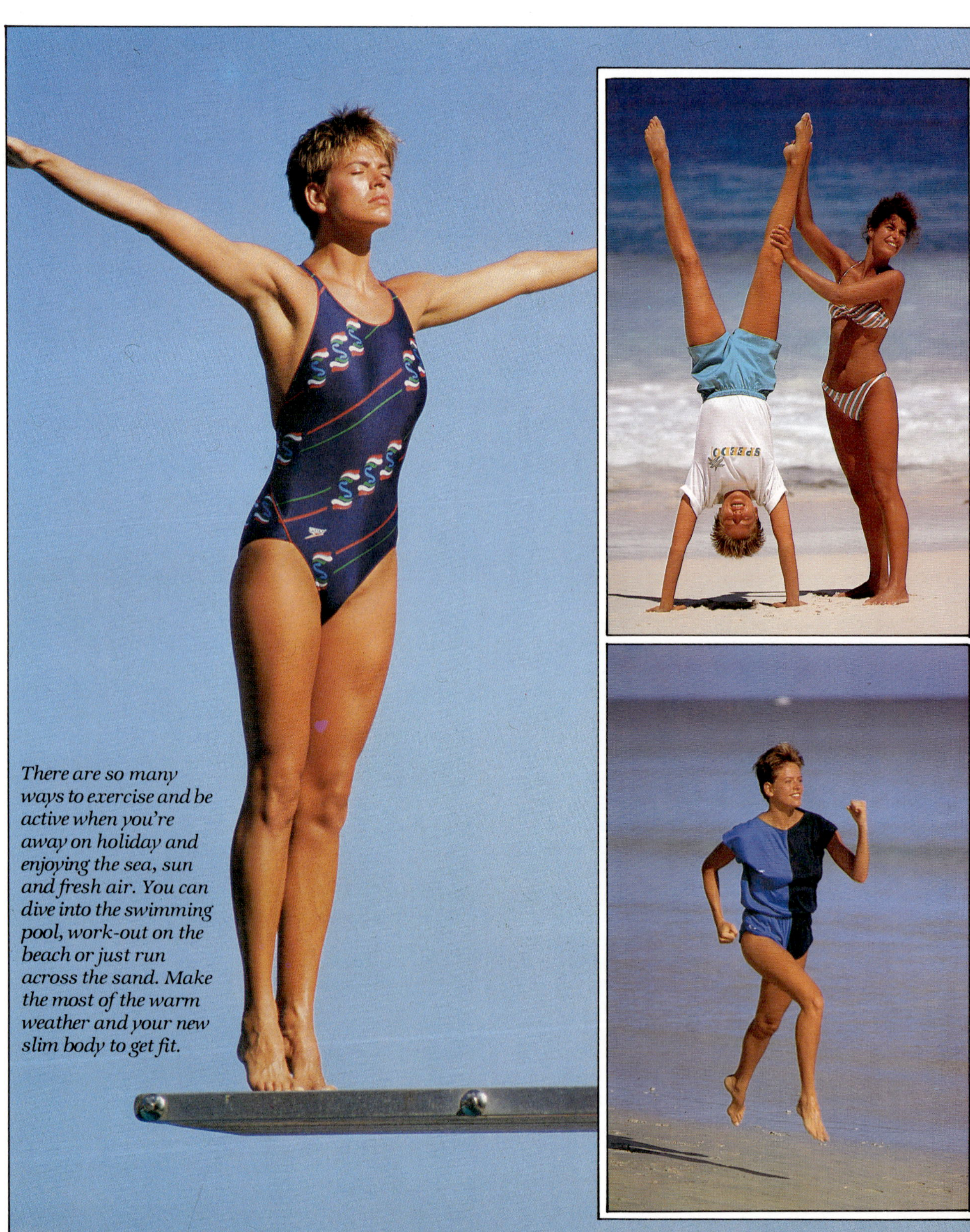

There are so many ways to exercise and be active when you're away on holiday and enjoying the sea, sun and fresh air. You can dive into the swimming pool, work-out on the beach or just run across the sand. Make the most of the warm weather and your new slim body to get fit.

Beach exercises with a difference

Don't just lie there on the beach — take advantage of the warm sunshine and have fun jogging through the foam at the water's edge or working-out with a beach towel. Not only will you feel fitter and more energetic but you will also get a better all-over tan if you keep on the move. Walking, running, swimming, beach games and watersports can all be part of your super holiday health plan. Exercise and the outdoor life are more enjoyable on holiday when you have plenty of time to spare and no worries about fitting them into a busy schedule.

Take the plunge

Opportunities for exercise are all around you, especially in the sea or swimming pool. Swimming uses your whole body, and is excellent for building up muscles, strengthening your heart and lungs and burning up calories to make you slimmer and more streamlined. If you make swimming part of your 28-day programme, you should be quite fit by the time you arrive at your holiday destination. Be sure to watch out for strong currents, and do not swim if red danger flags are flying or the lifeguards prohibit you from doing so. Respect for tides and currents is very important as swimming back to land may be more difficult than swimming out. Also, if you are in and out of the water all day, don't forget to keep reapplying a waterproof sunscreen.

If you don't feel like swimming, you can always work-out in the hotel pool. Use the swimming pool as your slimming pool. Because the water helps support your body, you are virtually weightless and you can exercise without straining joints and muscles.

Explore your surroundings

Be adventurous and discover the local countryside and coast by hiring a bicycle, putting on your running shoes or just walking. Cycling is a marvellous way of exercising muscles, burning up calories (about 600 per hour) and getting a good sun tan. You can hire bicycles in most resorts but check that the brakes are in good working order and the seat and handlebars adjusted to the correct height before you leave the hire centre. Look at the tyres to be sure that they are the right pressure and make sure the bike has a pump.

Running is the ideal holiday sport. You can do it any time and anywhere. All you need is some comfortable clothing and your running shoes and off you go — along the beach, up the cliff path, through the olive groves or across the fields. If it is very hot, then run only in the early morning before the sun's ultra-violet rays become intense, or in the evening when the heat of the day is subsiding. Running in hot midday sunshine may lead to dehydration and even sunstroke if you aren't careful.

Walking is another enjoyable way to explore, especially on cool summer evenings after a heavy dinner. Wear sensible low-heeled shoes, especially if you are clambering over sand-dunes and rocks.

Beach games

Use your time on the beach to the best advantage. After your 28-day programme your body should be in reasonably good shape, toned-up and looking good for summer's lighter and more revealing clothing. You can enjoy chasing a frisbee, exercising with a beach ball or working-out with a towel. You can even do a little weight-training, using cans of drink as dumb-bells. If you go with your family or make new friends on holiday, why not have a game of volleyball or hand-ball? Many beaches have a net rigged up for this purpose.

Many resorts have tennis courts where you can book a game, and there may be opportunities for more exciting sports like surfing, board-sailing, para-gliding or water skiing. Inquire at your hotel or ask the tour company's representative for details.

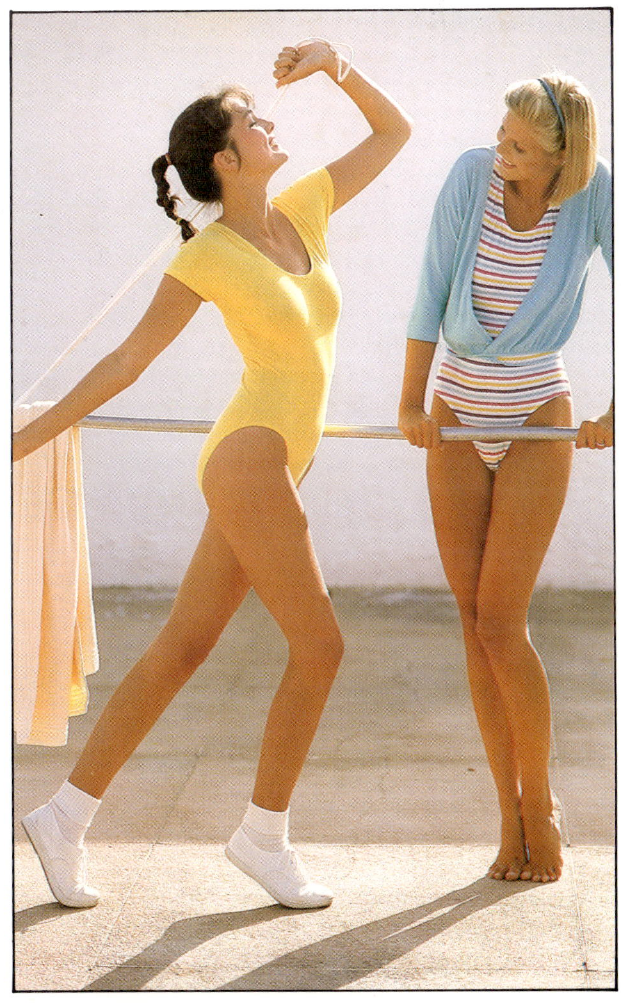

Holiday reference guide

More and more people are choosing to take their car on a motoring holiday and go touring in their own or another country. Wherever you're planning to go, it's very important that your car should be roadworthy and that you are prepared for the journey ahead.

1 Service your car

Two or three weeks before you plan to leave, you should book your car into a garage for a service. If you are mechanically minded, do it yourself. Your car will need to be reliable and in good working order for a long journey. Don't leave the service to the last minute — it may be necessary to order new parts and this sometimes takes time. Also, it's a good idea to run around in the car afterwards and give it time to settle down, just in case any work still needs to be done. You will need to check the following:

Brakes should be working efficiently. They may need renewing if they are well-worn. After all, they may be life-saving in an accident. Brake fluid should also be checked and topped up if necessary.

Tyres will need replacing if the tread is very worn — ask your garage for advice. Be sure to take a spare tyre in reasonable condition in case you have a puncture. Check the tyre pressures before you depart.

Lights should also be working properly. Find out from your motoring association if there is any special legislation governing their uses in the countries you plan to visit. For instance, sidelights may be needed even in daylight hours (in Sweden); or left-dipping headlights may not be permissible. And check that headlamps are adjusted to the right height.

Electrical systems should function as intended with no loose connections or faulty wiring. Check the battery acid levels and terminals. Make sure that the terminal leads to the battery are secured and not frayed. Your spark plugs may need replacing if your car has done over 10,000 miles since its last service.

Radiator water level should be checked — obviously, this does not apply to cars with sealed radiator systems. If you are driving through the mountains and high alpine passes, it may be a good idea to put in some anti-freeze.

Other things to be looked at include possible engine faults and strange noises or vibrations, the steering, clutch and gearbox, suspension and bodywork. Before you leave, do the following:

1 Top up the oil if necessary if levels are getting low.

2 Make sure that seat-belts are properly adjusted and working efficiently.

3 The rear view and side mirrors should be adjusted to the correct angle.

4 The roof rack should be attached properly and securely.

5 Windscreen wipers should be replaced if suspect. In doubt, take spares.

6 Give the car a good clean, paying special attention to the windscreen and rear window. Pack a chamois leather, some cloths and window-cleaning fluid in the boot before you go.

2 Useful items to take with you

On a motoring holiday, you may find that some of the following suggestions come in useful. Pack them in the car just in case.

Spares kit: all the usual spares (provided by motoring organisations) plus electrical cable, gasket sealing compound, insulating tape, inner tube, spare tyre, radiator sealing compound, hose, fan belt, distributor cap, fuses, bulbs, fuel-pump set, windscreen wipers.

Glove compartment: maps and car manual, torch, sunglasses, car compass, driving gloves, fire extinguisher, first aid kit.

Boot: tow-rope, flashing emergency lamp, warning triangle, windscreen de-mister, sponges, jack, spanners, screwdrivers, oil, hammer, wheel brace.

3 Insurance matters

You may need an international insurance certificate (green card) to ensure that whichever country you are driving through, you automatically have the same level of cover as you do at home. This can be obtained from your insurance company on request. All motoring insurance policies in EEC member countries together with some other European states extend to third party insurance, but you must check with your own insurance company to see what you are entitled to in the way of additional or comprehensive cover. Some motoring organisations run their own special insurance policies which cover cars of all ages. It may be worth taking out one of these.

4 Documents and licences

Your driving licence is valid in most countries although some require an International Driving Permit or an official translation of your licence, these are usually issued free of charge by your motoring association. You must also carry the vehicle registration book, and display a plate with GB or your country's initials on the back of your car or trailer. If driving in Spain, you are advised to take out a bail bond — your insurer can supply one. This guarantees that in the case of a road accident for which you are deemed by the authorities to be at fault, that money will be available to pay bail and prevent you being put into jail. If you are motoring in Eastern Europe you will need a *carnet.* Buy it from your motoring organisation before you set out. It will avoid any misunderstandings about the payment of import duty when you enter a country.

5 Motorail can make journeys easier
If you have a long way to drive, you might consider putting your car on the train to cross Europe. Then you can relax on the way and arrive at your destination or touring base refreshed and ready to enjoy your motoring holiday. Long hours spent on *autoroutes* and *autobahns* can be exhausting — the train will take all the hard work out of getting there and ensure that you start your holiday in the right frame of mind. However, it is not a cheap way to travel and you must compare the cost of motorail with a long drive and overnight hotel stops. A better way of cutting down travel time might be to fly out and back and hire a car while you tour around. There are many good fly-drive deals available from most tour operators.

6 Hiring a car
If you decide to hire a car abroad, you can either book before you leave the country with one of the large international hire companies or rent one at the airport when you arrive. It is probably better to hire in advance so that you can choose the car you want to drive and it can be ready waiting at the airport when you land. Before you drive it away, make sure that the car is in good working order and that you understand the controls and electrics. Check that brakes, lights, clutch and steering are OK. Look at the tyres to inspect the tread. Make sure that the window washers are full, the wipers work properly and that the horn and indicators function, too. You should also know how to open the petrol filler cap, bonnet and boot. If you're unhappy about the car, don't be afraid to complain and ask for another one. You don't want an accident to spoil your holiday and some firms require you to sign a statement that the car is in good working order before you drive it away. So make sure that it is. Also, check that the petrol tank is full. It would be awful to break down further down the road on an empty tank.

You will have to put down a deposit unless you pay by credit card for the car hire. If you pay a mileage rate, check the clock with the company's employee before you leave. To avoid possible fraud, don't sign a blank credit card voucher. Instead, estimate the amount that should be due and be prepared to pay any extra when you bring the car back. Check the conditions of hire and insurance cover carefully — your own comprehensive cover may not be applicable to a hire car.

7 Taking the car on a ferry
Car ferries operate on most routes between Britain and the Continent and are the usual way to take your car abroad. You can book on a boat or hovercraft (often a more bumpy ride). The summer peak holiday period is always busy, so book up in advance to ensure that you get the crossing and dates you want. At the same time, check that your insurance policy covers a sea crossing (most do). If you take a night crossing, it's a good idea to book a cabin so that you wake refreshed and ready to set off on a long drive.

8 Loading up the car
Start loading up the car the day before you leave. Make sure that you can get all the cases and other luggage in and try to distribute the weight evenly. Obviously, it is best to keep baggage as light as possible. A heavy car will eat up petrol, drive more slowly and may even affect the steering and handling. A roof-rack is useful, especially if the boot is small and you have several passengers. Strap any bags and cases down safely and cover with a waterproof sheet, also securely fastened to stop it flapping in high winds. Check that you have your spares kit and other useful items (see opposite) safely stowed aboard. Take a thermos flask, ice-box and some food for the journey.

9 Taking a caravan
Before you set out, make sure that the brakes are working properly, that the car wing mirrors are wide enough to give good vision behind the caravan and that the tow bracket is solid and secure. The indicators and brake lights on the back of the caravan should also be in good working order.

Pack everything carefully inside the caravan — breakable china should be made immoveable. Better still, make do with unbreakable plastic plates and tin mugs. Put any weighty items low down in the caravan to prevent its centre of gravity becoming too high. Stow everything securely and make sure that any cupboard doors are padlocked so that they can't burst open in transit.

If you are intending to tour, book up in advance for overnight stays at various sites — they are often mobbed in summer. You can get details of sites abroad and their amenities from tourist offices and travel agents.

10 Beating carsickness
The most obvious way to do this is to fly or sail to your destination, but lots of people suffer from this at some time or another. If you are inclined to do so, take some travel sickness pills before you set out. Drivers are less likely to feel sick than their passengers and they should be cautious about taking any medication which might induce drowsiness. In addition, don't eat any rich or fatty fried foods which might upset your stomach before driving. Some people find that a car with hard suspension is preferable to a more luxurious saloon which bounces along as though on a cushion.

If you are going abroad on holiday, you will need to take some foreign currency and travellers cheques with you. They can both be purchased over the counter in a bank or bureau de change. Even if you do not have a bank account, you can exchange cash for them. Although some large branches keep a stock of American dollars, French francs, Italian lire and other popular currencies, you will probably find that small branches have to order them specially so it is just as well to give your bank at least a week's notice to give them time to get in what you need. Of course, you can also exchange money at the airport if you are in a hurry.

Foreign currency

When you change your money, check on the current exchange rates as these vary literally from day to day. Expect to pay a commission which will be a percentage of the amount of foreign currency you buy. Although it is a good idea to have some loose change and banknotes on you when you arrive at your holiday destination, travellers cheques and credit cards are safer than cash. If you are robbed or lose your wallet, any cash is probably irrecoverable, but loss of credit cards can be notified to the issuing company so that you are not deemed liable for any subsequent purchases.

Travellers cheques

Order these from your bank. They can be changed abroad in most banks, bureaux de change and hotels for cash. Exchange rates vary so you will have to shop around for the best deal — often the most handy places to cash them, such as your hotel, are the most expensive. Banks usually give the best deal. You can also pay directly for your accommodation, meal or purchases in some hotels, restaurants and shops with travellers cheques as long as you have some form of identification with you, such as a passport or identification card with your photo attached. US dollar cheques are more widely accepted than other currencies. Be wary of any unofficial money changers, especially in the Far East. You may pay dearly for their services. When cashing cheques abroad, make sure that you are not short-changed. This is all too easy if you are not familiar with the currency and current exchange rates. Try and calculate in advance how many pesetas, dollars, lire or drachma you will get. In Italy you may even be handed packets of sweets and telephone tokens along with notes and coins in exchange.

Credit cards

This plastic money is very useful indeed when travelling. Most shops, hotels, restaurants and night-clubs accept credit cards from major banks and companies such as Barclaycard, American Express, Access and Diners Club. Because you don't have to pay straight away and are allowed at least a month's instant-free credit, they are a good way of handling your money. However, after the initial limit, interest charges are very high. In this way you can pay many of your holiday bills and expenses after you return home and not have to worry about carrying large amounts of money around with you. They can also bypass any foreign allowances that operate in some countries.

Banks abroad

Banking hours vary from country to country, although most banks are open in the mornings from Monday to Friday and often in the afternoons for a few hours, too. In some countries, they may even stay open at weekends and evenings for foreign exchange facilities only. When changing cash or travellers cheques in a bank, always remember to take your passport with you. Of course, not all banks will change your money and you may have to try several before you get lucky. In the United States in particular, very few banks, even in a large city like New York, have exchange facilities and so a credit card is more useful.

When you return home

It is always a good idea to keep your exchange receipts in order to satisfy any local currency regulations when leaving some countries. Any cash can be changed back into your own currency at the airport when you return home. Your bank will exchange notes and travellers cheques but not coins, so try to get rid of these at the airport or on the plane coming home. Use them to buy magazines and drinks, or put them away in a safe place for your next trip.

If you run out of money

Good management and advance planning should ensure that this does not happen to you. However, if you do run out of money, you can always arrange a bank transfer. All you need do is to contact your local bank manager by telex, phone or letter, letting him know the amount of money needed and why, the address to which it is to be sent and the method of dispatch. He can then transfer the money to the bank of your choice. Of course, this is an expensive and may be a lengthy business, so try not to let it happen to you. If you are going abroad for a long holiday, say, a couple of months, it might be worthwhile to arrange for special banking facilities at a bank abroad. Your bank at home will be able to arrange this for you before you leave. You just have to let them know exactly where you're going and ask for money to be transferred.

Adventure and activity holidays

If you are feeling really fit and energetic at the end of the programme, then some kind of activity holiday, especially a sports-orientated one, may be just right for you. There are many holidays to choose from which cover general leisure interests, ordinary sports and even more adventurous activities such as deep-sea diving, pot-holing, hang-gliding and parachuting. Here is a brief guide to some unusual holidays:

1 Adventure holidays

Under this heading, you can choose from ballooning, canoeing, caving, climbing, hang-gliding, flying and gliding, parachuting, sailing and diving holidays. For details of what is available, write to the relevant authority or sports body, or look through the specialist magazines for details and special offers. If you are a beginner or still relatively inexperienced, check that there is qualified instruction and that safety levels are high, especially in more dangerous sports like mountaineering. If you decide to go on one of these holidays, take out some form of personal insurance cover just to be on the safe side. National tourist offices for different countries should be able to supply leaflets and details of this sort of activity holiday.

Another exciting holiday is to go to Africa on safari and see the marvellous wildlife in its natural habitat. There are many packages available ranging from the luxurious to the rough-it variety. If you are getting back to nature, so to speak, you may prefer to camp out in a tent under the stars and cook your supper over a camp fire. However, most people prefer a few civilised comforts and even in the wilds of East Africa there are luxury hotels equipped with swimming pools and first-class restaurants to cater for their every need.

Overland holidays are also becoming popular, especially among young people. These are organised by many specialised travel companies and feature such faraway romantic places as Nepal, Tibet, India, the Middle East and Africa. Sometimes they include discount airfares. Now that the so-called hippy trail through Afghanistan has been closed due to Soviet intervention, it is almost impossible to travel overland all the way to the Far East and Asian subcontinent.

2 Sporting holidays

If you prefer to spend your holiday playing tennis, golf, squash or riding and pony-trekking, orienteering or surfing and water-skiing, there are many good offers with professional coaching thrown in. The advantage of this type of holiday is that you are doing something you enjoy with other like-minded people. It is easy to make friends who share the same interests and you won't get bored, especially if you are the sort of person who cannot lie in the sun for long periods at a stretch without wanting to get up and do something. Make sure that you get the sort of accommodation you want and can afford. Although some of these holidays are planned around first-class hotels, you may also have the option of farmhouses and guest houses (as on pony trekking holidays), self-catering villas, apartments and cottages, or even residential accommodation in a school or university during academic holidays. If you want to enjoy the sunshine at the same time, you may find a wide range of sporting offers in Spain and Portugal, especially if you like tennis or golf. In fact, the Algarve is often referred to as the 'Costa Golf'!

Skiers are well catered for with most travel tour operators running cheap packages in the winter months at European and American ski resorts. But if you would like to go skiing in summer, there are several resorts at very high altitudes where the snow is sufficiently good to ski all the year round. Ask your travel agent for further details and brochures.

3 Special interest holidays

These cater for more gentle pursuits such as arts and crafts, painting, birdwatching, drama, fishing, table-tennis and walking. Other interesting holidays include helping out on an archaeological dig or going to arts and music festivals. Walking holidays are a great way of seeing the countryside, getting fit and enjoying the open air in a more leisurely way. You can either join the Youth Hostels Association or Ramblers Association, and stay at special cheap hostels overnight, or carry a tent on your back, or even walk between country house hotels. The choice is yours.

4 Working holidays

Some people will even pay you to go on holiday as long as you work. There are special directories listing vacation opportunities for students, but you could also try fruit and grape picking in France; working on an Israeli kibbutz or in an American summer camp; teaching overseas or helping out on sporting holidays. If your haven't got much money you might earn enough in two or three weeks to pay for another week of travel or sunbathing before you return home. Browse through the books in your local reference library for details and addresses of where to apply.

5 Healthy holidays

If your idea of a holiday is just relaxing or getting fitter and trimmer and being generally self-indulgent, then a fortnight at a health farm may be just right for you. There are many of these throughout Europe and North America where you can go to top up your energy and recover from the rigours of a demanding career. Some are in sunny Mediterranean resorts so you can develop a glorious sun tan without any worries of putting on holiday weight through too much food and wine.

Holiday reference guide

Travelling by plane is not the glamorous or romantic experience it used to be — nowadays, international airports are busy, noisy places, and planes are often cramped and uncomfortable, especially on a long flight. If you have booked a holiday package, all you need do is check-in at the airport and then you will probably be well taken care of — shepherded onto the plane, through customs at the other end and whisked onto the coach that will transport you to your hotel. Travellers on scheduled and stand-by flights may face other difficulties — apart from the usual delays and cancellations, there may be overbooking of seats, for instance. However, there are a few things you can do to make getting away and your flight easier:

1 Getting to the airport
Your ticket or the travel itinerary provided by the tour operator or travel agent will clearly state the time by which you should check-in at the airport. Make sure that you have plenty of time to spare. Don't try to cut it fine and have a last-minute panic running onto the plane. Allow time for traffic jams, problems parking the car, train, coach or bus delays and for children, too, if you are taking them along. Many airports have special long-term carparks at reasonable rates but they are often some distance away and you may need to wait for a coach or minibus service to pick you up and take you to the departures terminal. Some private operators have security-patrolled carparks and will run you backwards and forwards to the airport to and from your flight.

2 At the airport
As soon as you arrive at the departures building you must check-in for your flight. In other words, you must go with your tickets and luggage to the airline counter where your flight number is shown. Here, your tickets are checked, your baggage is weighed and labelled and sets off on its separate journey down the conveyor belt to the plane. You will probably be allocated a seat number in a smoking or non-smoking area, and then you are free to wander off and change your money, buy some magazines or enjoy a coffee before going through passport control and into the departures lounge.

Once they have successfully negotiated passport control and the usual security checks, most people head for the duty free-shops. If you wish to buy some cheap goods you will have to show your ticket and boarding card at the check-out counter. Duty-free allowances vary throughout the world so check up on how much wine, spirits, cigarettes, tobacco or perfume you are allowed to take out with you, and back into the country when you return home.

You must wait in the departures lounge until your flight is called and then proceed to the correct departure gate for boarding. Your ticket and boarding card may be checked again before you enter the plane so keep them handy in an easily accessible place.

3 In-flight
You will be shown how to fasten your seat-belt and the safety procedures for the aircraft in which you are travelling. On take-off and landing and during bad patches of turbulence you will be asked to extinguish cigarettes and fasten seat-belts. Meals and entertainment on board vary a great deal, depending on flight time and whether you are travelling on an economy, club or first class ticket. If meals are available, as on longer hauls, you can ask in advance (when you book) for a special meal if you wish. Most major international airlines provide vegetarian, kosher, diabetic, low-calorie, fat-free, gluten-free, salt-free and Muslim food when requested.

Alcohol is available, too, on most flights — likewise soft drinks, tea and coffee. But these may not be free as of right. Quite often you have to pay for them, although at duty-free prices. On shorter flights, you may be given coffee and biscuits or a snack. Find out what is provided so that you can take some food with you if necessary, especially if you are flying with children. Remember, though, that it is prohibited to take fresh food into many countries, so you will have to eat it on the plane and not take it with you when you disembark.

Passing the time: on long flights, you may be able to purchase a headset and listen to the in-flight entertainment channels providing a variety of music and humour, or even watch a current feature film. Be prepared for the fact that sound quality is often poor — it is possible to see some films and understand about one word in ten! You can kill flying time by reading books, newspapers and magazines (sometimes provided by the airline), talking to your neighbours or playing games such as crosswords, quizes or cards. On a large aircraft, such as a jumbo, you can even walk around and stretch your legs. On major intenational and transcontinental flights, the staff usually open up a duty-free shop or wheel a trolley through the plane in case you didn't have time to purchase things at the airport.

Comfort: planes are notoriously uncomfortable, especially on a flight of three hours or more.

Although modern planes are pressurised, feet still tend to swell and ears may 'pop'. You may feel very hot or rather cold, depending on the temperature inside the cabin. Guard against this by travelling in loose cotton clothes. Take a warm jacket with you and a pair of slippers for long-distance flights. Don't wear tight shoes — you may not be able to get them on again when you deplane! If you experience pressure in your ears, try sucking a boiled sweet or swallowing hard and blowing your nose.

If you want to sleep to pass the time and make your journey pass more quickly, ask the stewardess for a pillow and blanket to make yourself more comfortable. These are usually handed out anyway on night flights and the main lights are switched off. You can always switch on your overhead reading light if you want to stay awake.

Fear of flying: many people are nervous or even very frightened indeed of flying yet statistics show that it is probably the safest method of travel, even if you might believe otherwise when you are high up in the blue yonder gazing down on banks of fluffy white clouds. Don't worry about such things as variations in engine noise, bumpiness and thunderstorms. You will hear particularly loud engine noise, especially on taking-off and landing. There may be a clunk as the undercarriage and wheels are neatly folded away or lowered. Often the pilot will warn you in advance of the noisy crescendo when the engine is put into reverse thrust on landing and the plane seems to career along the runway until it comes to a welcome halt near the end. Although flying through a thunderstorm is relatively safe, most pilots try to fly round them. They are told of their location through weather reports and radar — likewise for turbulence which is nothing to worry about but can be frightening for passengers when the plane bumps along spectacularly. Basically, the higher you fly, the less risk there is of encountering these bumpy patches of air. It's more likely in the first 20,000 feet, going through cloud and crossing mountains and coastlines. Don't be anxious — it's just a normal part of flying and nothing to worry about.

Sickness: a few unfortunate people suffer from airsickness. If you are one of these, then take a travel sickness pill in good time. Ask for a seat in the most stable part of the aircraft — preferably not in the tail end but in the main body of the plane. Keep your head as immobile as possible against the headrest on your seat. Don't drink any alcohol to 'settle your stomach' or 'calm your nerves' — this may irritate your stomach even more and make you really sick. Nor should you smoke, or eat rich, fried or fatty foods — something bland is best like milk or a banana. If you are pregnant, ask your doctor which are the best travel pills to take. Most airlines will not allow you to fly after the eighth month of pregnancy, anyway.

4 Disembarking

During the flight you will probably be required to fill out disembarkation forms and possibly customs declarations, too, which you will have to show to passport control or immigration officials when you land. Don't stand up the minute the plane touches down on the runway. Stay in your seat with your seat-belt securely fastened until the plane taxis to a halt and the seat-belt sign goes off. Although there's always a mad scramble to collect cabin baggage and get off the aircraft, you will probably find that it is easier and no slower in the long run to stand back and let the more impatient go, and then get off in a more leisurely manner. You may still have quite a long walk to passport control and baggage reclaim so try not to be too loaded up with hand luggage and duty-free goods.

If you are in transit and changing planes only then you probably won't have to go through passport control, but all other travellers must do so. Your passport may be stamped with the name of the airport and your date of arrival. If you have a visa, this will be checked to make sure that all is in order and you may be asked a few questions about the nature of your visit and how long you intend to stay. Having successfully negotiated passport control, it's time to pass on to the baggage reclaim hall to collect your cases. If you are lucky, they may already be there, but usually there is a wait before the first bag appears on the carousel. In the meantime, find a trolley on which to load your suitcases and be patient. When you spot your bags, check that they really are yours, especially if you have a chainstore case which may be identical to somebody else's.

Then pass on to customs. If you are arriving on holiday, you will probably not be asked for details of what you are bringing in. On your return journey home, however, you may be questioned about duty-free goods and gifts you bought abroad. Often there are two channels clearly labelled 'nothing to declare' and 'something to declare' — just go through the appropriate one into the arrivals area.

If you are on a package deal, the tour company's representative will probably be waiting to meet you and guide you to the coach which will take you to your hotel. Otherwise, there are always taxis or buses which operate between the airport and the nearest big city centre.

Index

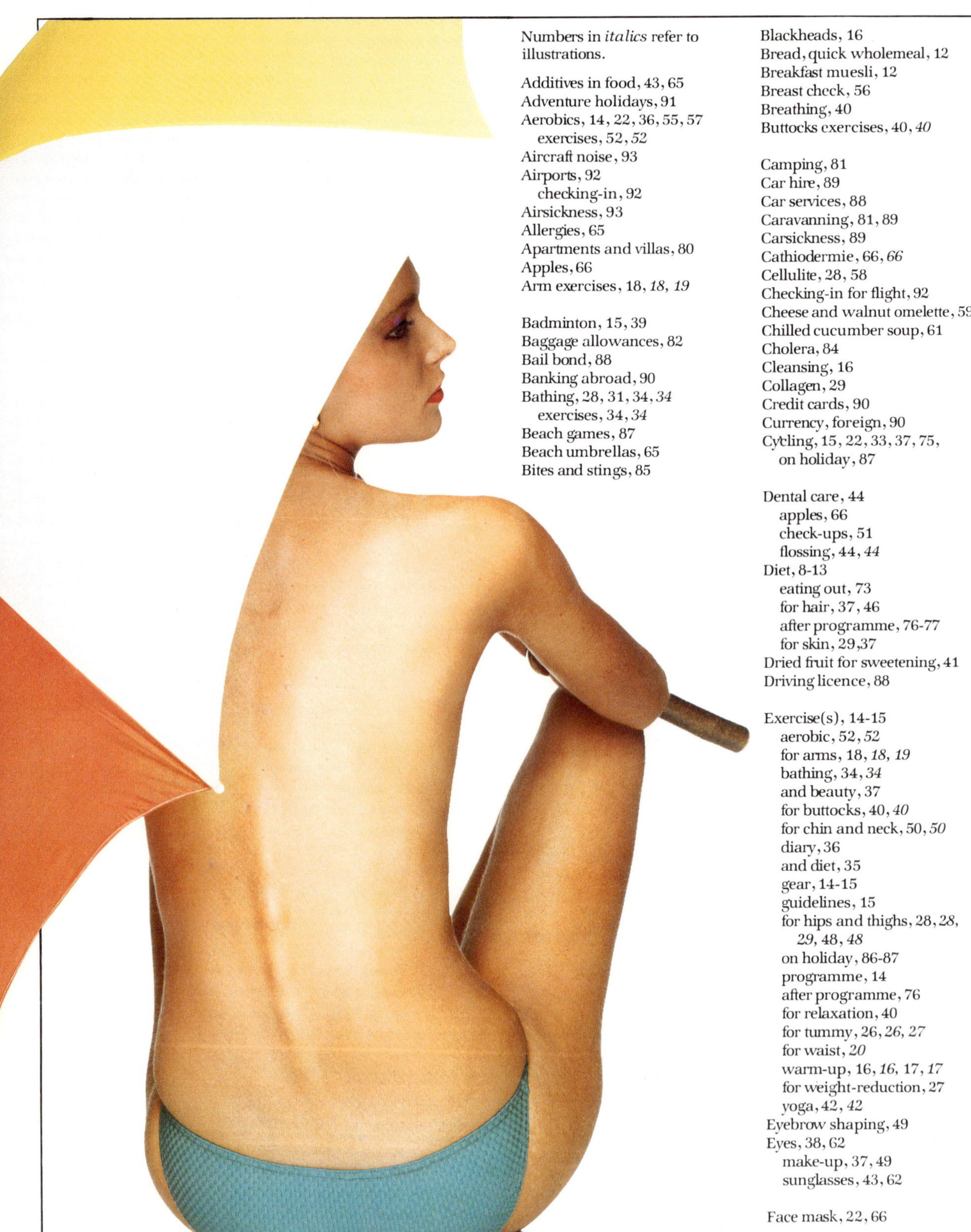

Numbers in *italics* refer to illustrations.

Additives in food, 43, 65
Adventure holidays, 91
Aerobics, 14, 22, 36, 55, 57
  exercises, 52, *52*
Aircraft noise, 93
Airports, 92
  checking-in, 92
Airsickness, 93
Allergies, 65
Apartments and villas, 80
Apples, 66
Arm exercises, 18, *18, 19*

Badminton, 15, 39
Baggage allowances, 82
Bail bond, 88
Banking abroad, 90
Bathing, 28, 31, 34, *34*
  exercises, 34, *34*
Beach games, 87
Beach umbrellas, 65
Bites and stings, 85
Blackheads, 16
Bread, quick wholemeal, 12
Breakfast muesli, 12
Breast check, 56
Breathing, 40
Buttocks exercises, 40, *40*

Camping, 81
Car hire, 89
Car services, 88
Caravanning, 81, 89
Carsickness, 89
Cathiodermie, 66, *66*
Cellulite, 28, 58
Checking-in for flight, 92
Cheese and walnut omelette, 59
Chilled cucumber soup, 61
Cholera, 84
Cleansing, 16
Collagen, 29
Credit cards, 90
Currency, foreign, 90
Cycling, 15, 22, 33, 37, 75,
  on holiday, 87

Dental care, 44
  apples, 66
  check-ups, 51
  flossing, 44, *44*
Diet, 8-13
  eating out, 73
  for hair, 37, 46
  after programme, 76-77
  for skin, 29,37
Dried fruit for sweetening, 41
Driving licence, 88

Exercise(s), 14-15
  aerobic, 52, *52*
  for arms, 18, *18, 19*
  bathing, 34, *34*
  and beauty, 37
  for buttocks, 40, *40*
  for chin and neck, 50, *50*
  diary, 36
  and diet, 35
  gear, 14-15
  guidelines, 15
  for hips and thighs, 28, *28, 29*, 48, *48*
  on holiday, 86-87
  programme, 14
  after programme, 76
  for relaxation, 40
  for tummy, 26, *26, 27*
  for waist, *20*
  warm-up, 16, *16*, 17, *17*
  for weight-reduction, 27
  yoga, 42, *42*
Eyebrow shaping, 49
Eyes, 38, 62
  make-up, 37, 49
  sunglasses, 43, 62

Face mask, 22, 66

Facial, 66, *66*
  sauna, 43
Fat-soluble vitamins, 19
Fats in diet, 53
Ferries, 89
Fibre, 8, 58
Flying, 92-93
  jet-lag, 74
  problems, 81
Footcare, 54, 62
  pedicure, *54*
Freckles, 35,
Fresh fruit fool, 77
Frittata, 37
Fruit,
  dried, 41
  in face masks, 22
  fool, fresh, 77
  growing your own, 61
  juices, 17, 22
  salad, summer, 29, *29*

Gazpacho, 25
Greek baked fish, 65
Greek salad, 17, *17*
Grilled kebabs, 23, *23*
Grilled salmon and
  avocado, 73, *73*

Hair, 46-47
  conditioning, 18, 26, 74
  cutting, 23, 46, 75
  damaged, 18
  dandruff, 18
  and diet, 33
  dry, 26
  dull, 18
  mousses for setting, *74*
  oily, 18, 26
  shampooing, 18, 74
  special effects, 46
  suncare, 46-47, 74
Hands, 62
  manicure, 24, *24*
Hangover, 85
Health farms, 91
Heat stroke, 84
Herbs, 23
  for beauty and health, 59
  in facial sauna, 43
Hip-slimming exercises,
  28, *28*, *29*
Hiring a car, 89
Holiday checklist, 78-80
Home-made yoghurt, 12
Hotels, 80
Hovercraft, 89

Insurance,
  for adventure holidays, 91
  medical, 29, 84
  motoring, 88
  travel, 29
Isotonics, 14

Jelly fish, 85
Jet-lag, 74
Jogging, 16, 20, 36
Juice(s),
  extractor, 17
  fruit, 17
  vegetable, 28

Kebabs,
  grilled, 23, *23*
  seafood, 41, *41*
Khoshaf, 53

Legs,
  cellulite, 58
  exercises for, 28, *28*, 29, *29*, *48*
  moisturising, 58
  shaving, 58
  varicose veins, 58
  waxing, 58
Lemon chicken, 55
Lips, 62
Luggage, 56, 82, *83*

Make-up, 62-63, 72, *72*
  for eyes, 49, *53*
  for sports, 37, 38
  10-minute routine, 53
Malaria, 84
Manicure, 24, *24*
Massage, 32, *32*
  for cellulite, 28
  for scalp, 64
  skin brushing, 61
Medical, 84-85
  health problems, 84-85
  insurance, 29, 84
  supplies, 48
  vaccination, 84
Mediterranean fish, 67, *67*
Mineral water, 21, 28
  and jet-lag, 74
Moisturising, 16, 21, 34, 58
Motorail, 89
Motoring holidays, 88-89
Muesli, breakfast, 12, 37

Packed lunches, 8
Packing, 77, 82
Pasta,
  and prawn creole, 51, *51*
  tagliatelle al tonno, 27, *27*
Pedicure, 54, *54*
Poliomyelitis, 84
Pool exercises, 44, *44*
Posture, 50
Pregnancy, 85
Processed foods, 28
Protein, 8, 29, 39
  pack for hair, 18, 26

Quick wholemeal bread, 12

Rabies, 85
Ratatouille, 57
Raw foods, 37
Relaxation exercises, 40
Rice and avocado salad, 39
Rice stuffed pepper, 33
Roller-skating, 15, 73
Room-running, 60
Running, 14, 16-17, 20, 36,
  50, 55, 57, 64, 73
  and beauty, 37
  on holiday, 87
  injuries, 64
  room-running, 60
  shoes, 64, *64*
  stair-running, 55
  training pulse rate, 36, *36*
  warm-up exercises, 16, *16*,
    17, *17*, *20*

Safaris, 91
Salad(s), 49
  beans in, 39
  dressing, yoghurt, 12
  Greek, 17
  Nicoise, 45
  rice and avocado, 39, *39*
  spinach, 21
  summer fruit, 29
  tomato and lentil, 43
Sauna, 27
  facial, 43
Scalp massage, 64
Sea urchins, 85
Seafood kebabs, 41, *41*
Skin-brushing, 61
Skincare, 16, 62
  chart, 16
  and diet, 29, 37
  dry skin, 16
  face masks, 22, 66
  facial, 66, *66*
    sauna, 43
  moisturising, 21
  normal skin, 16
  oily skin,, 16
  routine, 16
Skipping, 25, 33
Slimming, tips, 55
Smoked haddock kedgeree, 35, *35*
Smoking, 17
Soup(s)
  chilled cucumber, 61
  gazpacho, 33
Spices, 23
Spinach salad, 21
Sporting holidays, 91
Sports bra, 56, *56*
Sports clinic, 64
Spots and blemishes, 16
Sprouted beans, 39
Squash, 15, 39
Stool-stepping, 50
Stuffed tomato platter, 74, *74*
Sugar, 41
Summer fruit salad, 29
Sunburn, 31
Sunglasses, 43, 62
Sunscreens, 30, 31, 37
  for hair, 47
Sun-tanning, 21, 30-31, 58
Swimming, 14-15, 22, 33, 75, 87

Tagliatelle al tonno, 27, *27*
Tandoori chicken dip, 49
Tanning, 21, 30-31, 58
Tennis, 15, 39, 59, *59*
Thigh-reducing exercises, 28,
  28, *29*, 48, *48*
Tomato and lentil salad, 43
Toning, 16
Travellers cheques, 90
Tummy-toning exercises, 26, *26*, *27*
Turbulence in flight, 93
Typhoid, 84

Vaccination, 84
Vegetable(s),
  juices, 28
  growing your own, 61
Vitamin(s), 19
  A, 19, 29
  B, 19, 29, 33, 37, 39
  C, 17, 19, 29, 37, 39, 58
  chart, 19
  D, 19
  E, 19, 29, 58
  for hair, 33

Waist-slimming exercises, 20, *20*
Walking, 87
Warm-up exercises, 16, *16*,
  17, *17*, *20*
Water, mineral, 21, 28
Water-soluble vitamins, 19, 37
Waxing legs, 58
Weight training, 38, *38*, *39*
Wholemeal bread, quick, 12
Working holidays, 91
Work-out, 14, 15, 67, 75

Yellow fever, 84
Yoga, 14, 15, 42, *42*
Yoghurt,
  face mask, 22
  home-made, 12
  salad dressing, 12
Youth Hostels Association, 91

Zinc, 33, 57

Picture Credits

We would like to thank the following for their help in supplying photographs:

Almay: pages 13, 15
Ambre Solaire: pages 6, 70
Avon Cosmetics Ltd: pages 15, 36, 56-57
Barry Bullough: page 9
Burberrys Ltd: page 83
Christopher Barker: pages 42, 50
Clairol Appliances: pages 28, 54
Clarins (U.K.) Ltd: pages 49, 68
Daniel Galvin: page 77
Eden Vale: pages 13, 55, 74
Edward Billington (Sugars) Ltd: page 11
Elizabeth Arden: pages 38, 72
Gillette: page 6
Grayshott Hall: pages 10-11, 66, 70, 75
Helena Rubinstein: pages 2-3, 34, 35, 58, 63, 70, 94
Jackie Genova: pages 7, 14-15
Le Coq Sportif: pages 59, 65
L'Oréal: pages 46, 47, 63, 64, 67, 74, 79
Pasta Information Centre: pages 27, 51
Piz Buin: pages 30-31
Raleigh: pages 33, 75
Shades International: page 7
Slix Swimwear: pages 4, 5, 6
Speedo (Europe) Ltd: pages 62, 83, 86
Summer Orange Office: pages 11, 13
The Big Apple Health Studios: page 60, 76
Triumph International: pages 41, 56, 61, 71, 87
Tupperware: pages 12, 23, 35, 39, 67